Study Guide to Accompany

MEDICAL-SURGICAL NURSING

An Integrated Approach

2nd Edition

Lois White, RN, PhD

Former Chairperson, Professor
Department of Vocational Nurse Education
Del Mar College
Corpus Christi, Texas

Gena Duncan, RN, MS, MSEd

Asst. Professor and
Director of Associate Degree Program
University of Saint Francis
Fort Wayne, Indiana

Prepared by
Kathleen Peck Schaefer, RNC, MSN, MEd
Clinical Instructor, Adjunct Faculty
School of Nursing
Marymount University
Arlington, Virginia
and
Nursing Staff
Inova Fairfax Hospital
Falls Church, Virginia

DELMAR

THOMSON LEARNING™   Australia   Canada   Mexico   Singapore   Spain   United Kingdom   United States

NOTICE TO THE READER

Publisher does not warrant or guarantee any of the products described herein or perform any independent analysis in connection with any of the product information contained herein. Publisher does not assume, and expressly disclaims, any obligation to obtain and include information other than that provided to it by the manufacturer.

The reader is expressly warned to consider and adopt all safety precautions that might be indicated by the activities herein and to avoid all potential hazards. By following the instructions contained herein, the reader willingly assumes all risks in connection with such instructions. The Publisher makes no representation or warranties of any kind, including but not limited to the warranties of fitness for particular purpose or merchantability, nor are any such representations implied with respect to the material set forth herein, and the publisher takes no responsibility with respect to such material. The publisher shall not be liable for any special, consequential, or exemplary damages resulting, in whole or part, from the readers' use of, or reliance upon, this material.

Delmar Staff:
Health Care Publishing Director: William Brottmiller
Executive Editor: Cathy L. Esperti
Acquisitions Editor: Matthew Filimonov
Senior Developmental Editor: Elisabeth F. Williams
Editorial Assistant: Melissa Longo
Executive Marketing Manager: Dawn F. Gerrain
Channel Manager: Tara Carter
Project Editor: Maureen M. E. Grealish
Production Coordinator: Anne R. Sherman
Senior Art/Design Coordinator: Timothy J. Conners

ISBN 0-7668-2568-X

Printed in the United States of America
1 2 3 4 5 6 7 8 9 10 XXX 05 04 03 02 01

For more information, contact Delmar, 3 Columbia Circle, PO Box 15015, Albany, NY 12212-0515; or find us on the World Wide Web at http://www.delmar.com

International Division List

Asia
Thomson Learning
60 Albert Street, #15-01
Albert Complex
Singapore 189969
Tel: 65 336 6411
Fax: 65 336 7411

Japan:
Thomson Learning
Palaceside Building 5F
1-1-1 Hitotsubashi, Chiyoda-ku
Tokyo 100 0003 Japan
Tel: 813 5218 6544
Fax: 813 5218 6551

Australia/New Zealand:
Nelson/Thomson Learning
102 Dodds Street
South Melbourne, Victoria
3205
Australia
Tel: 61 39 685 4111
Fax: 61 39 685 4199

UK/Europe/Middle East
Thomson Learning
Berkshire House
168-173 High Holborn
London
WC1V 7AA United Kingdom
Tel: 44 171 497 1422
Fax: 44 171 497 1426

Thomas Nelson & Sons LTD
Nelson House
Mayfield Road
Walton-on-Thames
KT12 5PL United Kingdom
Tel: 44 1932 2522111
Fax: 44 1932 246574

Latin America:
Thomson Learning
Seneca, 53
Colonia Polanco
11560 Mexico D.F. Mexico
Tel: 525-281-2906
Fax: 525-281-2656

Canada:
Nelson/Thomson Learning
1120 Birchmount Road
Scarborough, Ontario
Canada M1K 5G4
Tel: 416-752-9100
Fax: 416-752-8102

Spain:
Thomson Learning
Calle Magallanes, 25
28015-MADRID
ESPAÑA
Tel: 34 91 446 33 50
Fax: 34 91 445 62 18

International Headquarters:
Thomson Learning
International Division
290 Harbor Drive, 2nd Floor
Stamford, CT 06902-7477
Tel: 203-969-8700
Fax: 203-969-8751

Library of Congress Catalog Number: 2001028702

Contents

Preface..v

Acknowledgments vii

SECTION 1   FOUNDATIONS OF NURSING

UNIT 1   Factors Affecting Nursing Care

Chapter 1 The Health Care Delivery System 1

Chapter 2 Critical Thinking.......................7

Chapter 3 Legal Responsibilities 13

Chapter 4 Ethical Responsibilities............19

UNIT 2   Holistic Nursing Care

Chapter 5 Communication 25

Chapter 6 Cultural Diversity and Nursing..31

Chapter 7 Wellness Concepts 37

Chapter 8 Alternative/Complementary Therapies 41

Chapter 9 Loss, Grief, and Death............47

SECTION 2   AREAS OF MEDICAL-SURGICAL NURSING CARE

UNIT 3   Basic Concepts of Medical-Surgical Nursing

Chapter 10 Fluid, Electrolyte, and Acid–Base Balance....................................53

Chapter 11 IV Therapy 61

Chapter 12 Health Assessment 67

Chapter 13 Diagnostic Tests....................75

Chapter 14 Pain Management 83

Chapter 15 Anesthesia...........................91

Chapter 16 Nursing Care of the Surgical Client...97

Chapter 17 Nursing Care of the Oncology Client 105

UNIT 4   Oxygenation and Perfusion

Chapter 18 Nursing Care of the Client: Respiratory System 111

Chapter 19 Nursing Care of the Client: Cardiovascular System.............................121

Chapter 20 Nursing Care of the Client: Hematologic and Lymphatic Systems.........131

UNIT 5   Body Defenses

Chapter 21 Nursing Care of the Client: Integumentary System.............................139

Chapter 22 Nursing Care of the Client: Immune System.......................................147

Chapter 23 Nursing Care of the Client: HIV and AIDS..153

UNIT 6   Control, Mobility, Coordination, and Regulation

Chapter 24 Nursing Care of the Client: Musculoskeletal System 159

Chapter 25 Nursing Care of the Client:
Neurological System 167

Chapter 26 Nursing Care of the Client:
Sensory System......................................177

Chapter 27 Nursing Care of the Client:
Endocrine System 185

UNIT 7   Digestion and Elimination

Chapter 28 Nursing Care of the Client:
Gastrointestinal System 193

Chapter 29 Nursing Care of the Client:
Urinary System 201

**UNIT 8   Reproductive and
Sexual Disorders**

Chapter 30 Nursing Care of the Client:
Female Reproductive System 209

Chapter 31 Nursing Care of the Client:
Male Reproductive System........................217

Chapter 32 Nursing Care of the Client:
Sexually Transmitted Diseases 223

**UNIT 9   Physical and Mental
Integrity**

Chapter 33 Nursing Care of the Client:
Mental Illness...229

Chapter 34 Nursing Care of the Client:
Substance Abuse 237

**UNIT 10   Special Areas of
Medical-Surgical Nursing**

Chapter 35 Nursing Care of the
Older Client..243

Chapter 36 Rehabilitation, Home Health,
Long-term Care, and Hospice....................249

UNIT 11   Integration of Body Systems

Chapter 37 Nursing Care of the Client:
Responding to Emergencies 255

Chapter 38 Critical Thinking on
Multiple Systems.....................................261

Answer Key...267

Preface

This Study Guide is designed to accompany *Medical-Surgical Nursing: An Integrated Approach,* 2nd Edition, by Lois White and Gena Duncan. Each of the 38 chapters in this guide was created to facilitate student learning and refine student skills. By using this guide at home and in the clinical setting you will work with important concepts and begin to apply them to real-life situations.

To facilitate your learning, the chapters of this guide all include the following components:

- *Key Terms:* matching exercises designed to enhance your understanding of new terms presented in the text.
- *Abbreviation Review:* excercises to test your knowlege of abbreviations, acronyms, and symbols used in the text.
- *Exercises and Activities:* short scenarios with related questions to test your understanding and application of concepts.
- *Self-Assessment Questions:* multiple choice questions that draw on the key ideas in the chapter and prepare you to succeed in your examinations.

Acknowledgments

From the Author:

I want to thank my husband, Rusty, and son, Jeff, for their unfailing encouragement and support, which was so important to me while working on this project. To JoAnn, friend and colleague, your help was much appreciated. To Lois White and Gena Duncan, it has been my privilege to work on this project. Finally, to Beth Williams and Melissa Longo at Delmar, thanks for keeping me on track, for all the kind words, and for your editing expertise.

The Health Care Delivery System

Key Terms

Match the following terms with their correct definitions.

___ 1. Capitated Rate

a. Simultaneous existence of more than one disease process within an individual.

___ 2. Comorbidity

b. System of providing and monitoring care wherein access, cost, and quality are controlled before or during delivery of services.

___ 3. Exclusive Provider Organization

c. Care focused on promoting wellness and preventing illness.

___ 4. Fee for Service

d. Preset fee based on membership rather than services provided; payment system used in managed care.

___ 5. Health Care Delivery System

e. Organization wherein care must be delivered by the plan in order for clients to receive reimbursement for health care services.

___ 6. Health Maintenance Organization

f. Health care provider whom a client sees first for health care, typically a family practitioner (physician/nurse), internist, or pediatrician.

___ 7. Managed Care

g. Predetermined rate paid for each episode of hospitalization based on the client's age and principal diagnosis and the presence or absence of surgery or comorbidity.

___ 8. Medical Model

h. Health care delivery model wherein the government is the only entity to reimburse.

___ 9. Preferred Provider Organization

i. Prepaid health plan that provides primary health care services for a preset fee and focuses on cost-effective treatment methods.

___10. Prescriptive Authority

j. System in which the health care recipient directly pays the provider for services as they are provided.

___11. Primary Care

k. Traditional approach to health care wherein the focus is on treatment and cure of disease.

___12. Primary Care Provider

l. Legal recognition of the ability to prescribe medications.

___13. Primary Health Care

m. Care focused on diagnosis and treatment after the client exhibits symptoms of illness.

___14. Prospective Payment

n. Client's point of entry into the health care system; includes assessment, diagnosis, treatment, coordination of care, education, preventive services, and surveillance.

___15. Secondary Care

o. Mechanism for providing services that meet the health-related needs of individuals.

___16. Single-Payer System

p. Type of managed care model wherein member choice is limited to providers within the system.

___17. Single Point of Entry

q. A common feature of HMOs wherein the client is required to enter the health care system through a point designated by the plan.

___18. Tertiary Care

r. Care focused on restoring the client to the state of health that existed before the development of an illness; if unattainable, then care directed to attaining the optimal level of health possible.

Abbreviation Review

Write the definition of the following abbreviations and acronyms.

1. ADAMHA _____

2. AHCPR _____

3. AIDS _____

4. AMA _____

5. ANA _____

6. APRN _____

7. ATSDR _____

8. CCU _____

9. CDC _____

10. CHIP _____

11. CNM _____

12. CNO _____

13. CNS _____

14. CT _____

15. DDS _____

16. DMD _____

17. DRG _____

18. ECG _____

19. ED _____

20. EEG _____

21. EMG _____

22. EPO _____

23. FDA _____
24. HCFA _____
25. HIV _____
26. HMO _____
27. HRSA _____
28. ICU _____
29. IHS _____
30. JCAHO _____
31. LP/VN _____
32. MD _____
33. MRI _____
34. NCSBN _____
35. NFLPN _____
36. NIH _____
37. NLN _____
38. NP _____
39. OR _____
40. OT _____
41. PA _____
42. PCP _____
43. PPO _____
44. PT _____
45. RD _____
46. RN _____
47. RPCH _____
48. RPh _____
49. RR _____
50. RT _____
51. SBC _____
52. SW _____
53. USDHHS _____
54. USPHS _____
55. VA _____

Exercises and Activities

1. Which therapy departments or support services might be involved in the hospital setting for each of the following clients?
    a. A client who was recently diagnosed with diabetes: _____
    _____

    b. A client who requires extensive physical rehabilitation: _____
    _____

    c. A client diagnosed with a life-threatening illness: _____
    _____

2. a. What factors have contributed to the increased number of clients now receiving care in outpatient clinics and in home settings?
    _____
    _____
    _____

    b. Groups that are often unable to obtain adequate health care include: _____
    _____

3. Explain how the trends in health care are changing the practice of the LP/VN in relation to:

    a. Educational preparation for LP/VN licensure: _____
    _____

    b. Practice settings: _____
    _____

    c. Client population:
    _____
    _____

4. Mrs. Jacob is a 69-year-old client in your long-term care facility. She was admitted 2 weeks ago to continue her recovery from a hip fracture. Prior to her injury, she had been living alone in a small apartment in a retirement community not far from her married daughter. She has rejected her family's offer to move to their home but is now willing to accept some help with cleaning and cooking if it allows her to remain independent.

    List activities or referrals for Mrs. Jacob that would be examples of each level of care.

    Primary care: _____
    _____

    Secondary care: _____
    _____

    Tertiary care: _____
    _____

Self-Assessment Questions

Circle the letter that corresponds to the best answer for each question.

1. While participating in an immunization clinic, the nurse is providing
    a. primary care.
    b. secondary care.
    c. tertiary care.
    d. early intervention.

2. The system for financing health care services in the United States is based on
    a. a single-payer system.
    b. a managed-care model.
    c. an exclusive-provider model.
    d. a private insurance model.

3. The primary goal of managed care is to
    a. provide preventive services by a primary care provider.
    b. deliver service in the most cost-efficient manner possible.
    c. provide health education and disease prevention services to clients.
    d. set fees and determine reasonable reimbursement for medical and surgical treatment.

4. Conducting research and education related to specific diseases is a function of the
    a. National Institutes of Health.
    b. Centers for Disease Control and Prevention.
    c. Agency for Health Care Policy and Research.
    d. Health Resources and Services Administration.

5. The nurse providing care in the hospital setting knows that as a result of the Prospective Payment System and DRGs
    a. clients may be discharged sooner.
    b. clients are less likely to be critically ill.
    c. clients are receiving higher-quality care.
    d. clients' response to treatment is less important.

6. A major challenge facing the U.S. health care system is the
    a. greater availability of outpatient facilities and services.
    b. lack of prescriptive authority for advanced practice nurses.
    c. decreased use of hospitals and its impact on quality of care.
    d. cultural beliefs of a diverse population and their effect on health care.

Critical Thinking

Key Terms

Match the following terms with their correct definitions.

___ 1. Concept	a. To prove or show to be valid.
___ 2. Critical Thinking	b. Use of the elements of thought to solve a problem or settle a question.
___ 3. Discipline	c. Mode of thinking—about any subject, content, or problem—whereby the thinker improves the quality of his or her thinking by skillfully taking charge of the structures inherent in thinking and imposing intellectual standards (or a level of degree of quality) upon them.
___ 4. Disciplined	d. Branch of learning, field of study, or occupation requiring specialized knowledge.
___ 5. Judgment	e. Level or degree of quality.
___ 6. Justify	f. Mental picture of an abstract phenomenon that serves to organize observations related to that phenomenon.
___ 7. Logic	g. Trained by instruction and exercise.
___ 8. Opinion	h. Formal principles of a branch of knowledge (such as nursing).
___ 9. Reasoning	i. Introspective.
___ 10. Reflective	j. Conclusions that are based on sound reasoning and can be supported by evidence.
___ 11. Standard	k. Subjective belief.

Abbreviation Review

Write the meaning or definition of the following acronym.

1. UIS _____

Exercises and Activities

1. a. How will critical thinking skills help you as a student?

    _____

    _____

    _____

    b. In what ways will critical thinking help you provide expert nursing care?

    _____

    _____

    _____

    c. How would you explain the term "critical thinking" to another student?

    _____

    _____

    _____

2. Complete the following statements.
    a. To use the nursing process effectively, you must develop the skills of _____.
    b. Ideas or things taken for granted are called _____.
    c. The answer to a question that began a process of reasoning is called a _____.
    d. A person's _____ is based on many factors that develop a unique way of thinking and a unique perspective.
    e. The traits of a disciplined thinker include _____
    _____.

3. Identify techniques that can improve your thinking ability in each of the following areas.

    a. List three tactics that will help you to develop your reading skills.
    (1) _____
    (2) _____
    (3) _____

    b. State three techniques to improve your ability to write your thoughts clearly.
    (1) _____
    (2) _____
    (3) _____

    c. Write two questions that you can ask yourself to improve your listening skills.
    (1) _____
    (2) _____

    d. Identify two activities to improve your public speaking ability.
    (1) _____
    (2) _____

4. Your instructor has asked you to read the following paragraph from Chapter 1 and summarize the views of the writer to your classmates:

Greed and waste have been identified as major problems of the U.S. health care system. Whether these problems are caused by defensive practice, consumer demand, or professional economics is irrelevant to the public. Success in reform depends on starting where the public expects reform should begin: eliminating the greed of providers and the waste in the health care system. Further, people in the United States have become suspicious of health care providers. The high level of esteem in which medicine has traditionally been held has eroded over the past few years. Consumers, increasingly tired of paying the high cost of care, are questioning medical practices and fees. However, the public is not disillusioned with nurses. As reported in the AJN, a November 1999 Gallup poll reported that almost ¾ of those surveyed rated the honesty and ethics of nurses as "high" or "very high." Nurses received higher ratings than any other profession including other health care professionals. . . . Another survey . . . revealed that 92% of the public trust health information provided by registered nurses. This positive perception of nurses will be important as patterns of reform are established.

a. What important issue (or issues) is this writer addressing?

_____

_____

_____

b. How will you summarize the views of this writer for your classmates?

_____

_____

_____

c. If the writer came to your class, what additional questions might you want to ask?

_____

_____

_____

d. What questions might you anticipate from your classmates? From a group of physicans?

_____

_____

_____

5. The nurse in charge of your medical unit has mentioned to you that she would like to get some ideas on how to improve the support for new LP/VNs coming to work on the unit. Although a 4-week orientation program seems to help at first, many new LP/VNs leave the unit for other positions after only a few months or a year or two. Some nurses have said the pay isn't high enough, but you know nurses who have left the unit for lower-paying jobs, so that isn't the whole answer. Although retention is a complex problem, your nurse manager hopes you will come up with some ideas that can be implemented right away.

a. What is the main issue?

_____

_____

b. What do you need to know about this problem?

_____

_____

_____

c. You decide to form a small group to work with you on finding the causes and possible solutions. How will you select other people to work on this committee?

_____

_____

_____

d. What types of information will your committee need to collect for a thorough investigation of this issue?

_____

_____

_____

e. When you have completed your task, how will you clearly present the findings and suggestions to the nurse manager and your unit?

_____

_____

_____

f. How will critical thinking skills be involved throughout this process?

_____

_____

_____

Self-Assessment Questions

Circle the letter that corresponds to the best answer for each question.

1. All reasoning is based on using the skills of
    a. inferences.
    b. critical thinking.
    c. decision making.
    d. concept formation.

2. Anyone can work toward becoming a better thinker by developing
    a. specific attitudes, traits, and skills.
    b. introspective thinking techniques.
    c. opinions based on sound reasoning.
    d. philosophy statements related to nursing.

3. Students may improve their critical listening skills by
   a. requesting a bibliography.
   b. taking word-for-word notes.
   c. focusing on the mannerisms of the speaker.
   d. carrying on a mental dialogue with the speaker.

4. All reasoning is an attempt to
   a. problem solve.
   b. define concepts.
   c. determine assumptions.
   d. develop personal values.

5. Which statement is an example of an assumption?
   a. The minority population in the United States is growing every year.
   b. Women are better caretakers of children than are men.
   c. Clients want to be comfortable and free of pain.
   d. Elderly clients are better off at home.

6. A client wants to go home early from the hospital, saying, "My family can take better care of me at home than you can here." It is most important for the nurse to consider
   a. her personal biases.
   b. the patient's diagnosis.
   c. home health care nursing.
   d. the implications or consequences.

7. A nurse evaluates a client as overreacting to pain based on her own reaction to pain. This would be an example of
   a. empathy.
   b. reasoning.
   c. an inference.
   d. personal bias.

Legal Responsibilities

Key Terms

Match the following terms with their correct definitions.

___ 1. Administrative Law

    a. Civil wrong committed by a person against another person or property.

___ 2. Advance Directive

    b. Wrong that results from a deliberate deception intended to produce unlawful gain.

___ 3. Assault

    c. A legal document designating who may make health care decisions for a client when that client is no longer capable of decision making.

___ 4. Battery

    d. Law developed by those persons who are appointed to governmental administrative agencies and who are entrusted with enforcing the statutory laws passed by the legislature.

___ 5. Civil Law

    e. Contract that recognizes a relationship between parties for services.

___ 6. Confidential

    f. Obligation one has incurred or might incur through any act or failure to act.

___ 7. Constitutional Law

    g. Written instruction for health care that is recognized under state law and is related to the provision of such care when the individual is incapacitated.

___ 8. Contract Law

    h. Situation wherein a person is made to wrongfully believe that he cannot leave a place.

___ 9. Criminal Law

    i. Negligent acts on the part of a professional; relates to the conduct of a person who is acting in a professional capacity.

___10. Defamation

    j. Statute that is enacted by the legislature of a state and that outlines the scope of nursing practice in that state.

___11. Durable Power of Attorney for Health Care

    k. Enforcement of duties and rights among individuals and independent of contractual agreements.

13

___12. Expressed Contract

l. Law that provides protection to health care providers by ensuring them immunity from civil liability when care is provided at the scene of an emergency and the caregiver does not intentionally or recklessly cause the client injury.

___13. False Imprisonment

m. Enforcement of agreements among private individuals.

___14. Felony

n. Threat to do something that may cause harm or be unpleasant to another person.

___15. Formal Contract

o. Written contract that cannot be changed legally by an oral agreement.

___16. Fraud

p. A competent client's ability to make health care decisions based on full disclosure of the benefits, risks, potential consequences of a recommended treatment plan, and alternate treatments, including no treatment, and the client's agreement to the treatment as indicated by the client's signing a consent form.

___17. Good Samaritan Law

q. Risk-management tool used to describe and report any unusual event that occurs to a client, visitor, or staff member.

___18. Impaired Nurse

r. Law that deals with an individual's relationship to the state.

___19. Implied Contract

s. Guidelines established to direct nursing care.

___20. Incident Report

t. Unauthorized or unwanted touching of one person by another.

___21. Informed Consent

u. Law concerning acts of offense against the welfare or safety of the public.

___22. Law

v. Crime of a serious nature that is usually punishable by imprisonment in a state penitentiary or by death.

___23. Liability

w. Conditions and terms of a contract given in writing by the concerned parties.

___24. Libel

x. Law that deals with relationships between individuals.

___25. Living Will

y. Offense that is less serious than a felony and may be punished by a fine or by sentence to a local prison for less than 1 year.

___26. Malpractice

z. Words that are communicated verbally to a third party and that harm or injure the personal or professional reputation of another.

___27. Misdemeanor

aa. Law enacted by legislative bodies.

___28. Negligence

bb. Written words that harm or injure the personal or professional reputation of another person.

___29. Nursing Practice Act

cc. Private or secret.

___30. Peer Assistance Program

___31. Privacy

___32. Public Law

___33. Restraint

___34. Slander

___35. Standard of Practice

___36. Statutory Law

___37. Tort

___38. Tort Law

dd. Nurse who is habitually intemperate or is addicted to the use of alcohol or habit-forming drugs.

ee. Use of words to harm or injure the personal or professional reputation of another person.

ff. Rehabilitation program that provides an impaired nurse with referrals, professional and peer counseling support groups, and assistance and monitoring back into nursing.

gg. That which is laid down or fixed.

hh. Law that defines and limits the power of government.

ii. Any device used to restrict movement.

jj. General term referring to careless acts on the part of an individual who is not exercising reasonable or prudent judgment.

kk. Legal document that allows a person to state preferences about the use of life-sustaining measures should she be unable to make her wishes known.

ll. The right to be left alone, to choose care based on personal beliefs, to govern body integrity, and to choose when and how sensitive information is shared.

Abbreviation Review

Write the definition of the following abbreviations and acronyms.

1. ADA _____

2. ADA _____

3. AMA _____

4. AMA _____

5. ANA _____

6. CPR _____

7. DNR _____

8. DPAHC _____

9. HIV _____

10. IM _____

11. JCAHO _____

12. LP/VN _____

13. NCLEX _____

14. NFLPN _____

15. NPO _____

16. po _____

17. RN _____

Exercises and Activities

1. Give examples of how each of the following may directly affect your practice as an LP/VN.

   a. Statutory law: _____

   _____

   b. Administrative law: _____

   _____

   c. Contract law: _____

   _____

   d. Good Samaritan Act: _____

   _____

   e. Nursing practice act: _____

   _____

2. Match each situation with the probable type of tort involved.
   a. Assault and battery
   b. False imprisonment
   c. Invasion of privacy
   d. Defamation, libel
   e. Defamation, slander
   f. Negligence
   g. Malpractice

   _____ A student nurse is overheard talking in the cafeteria with fellow students about a client, Mr. Johnson, and his recent bout of depression.
   _____ A nurse asks a client why she chose Dr. Smith for her physician, saying, "He treats his patients like they were children, and is always so rude to the staff."
   _____ The nurse caring for a client with a new leg cast fails to routinely check the foot for adequate circulation. The client requires additional treatment and loses some function as a result.
   _____ The nurse is preparing to administer an intravenous antibiotic to the client. Because of a failure to check the armband, the wrong client receives the medication.
   _____ The nurse misreads an order for "2u of insulin" as "20 units of insulin" resulting in harm to the client.
   _____ A nurse fails to obtain an order for restraints that were initiated on a client who had become confused.
   _____ A client is told he must pay the remainder of his medical bill before he can leave the facility.
   _____ The names of the clients in a hospital unit are displayed on an assignment board.
   _____ Although the client is showing signs of an adverse reaction to a medication, the physician orders the medication to be continued. The nurse follows the physician's order.

3. Describe correct documentation in terms of timing of the entries, legibility, and thoroughness.

    _____

    _____

    a. In what ways can documentation support a nurse's actions?

    _____

    _____

4. What is the difference between a durable power of attorney for health care and a living will?

    _____

    _____

    a. Describe in your own words what you might include in your own health care directive or living will. Who would you designate to make health care decisions? What treatments would you want to have withheld?

    _____

    _____

    _____

5. Mr. Leonard is being treated for a fracture of his right hip. The nurse assigned to care for him is reviewing his chart for information. Because there is no advance directive, the nurse asks Mr. Leonard if he would like information or assistance to complete one. Mr. Leonard is uncomfortable and tells the nurse to let his wife sign any papers because she is the one who would make the decisions anyway.

    a. How could you explain an advance directive to Mr. Leonard and his wife? Can his wife sign the forms for him?

    _____

    _____

    b. Mr. Leonard is scheduled for surgery and the nurse is asked to witness the surgical consent form. In what circumstances should the nurse refuse to witness the form?

    _____

    _____

    c. The nurse believes that Mr. Leonard does not understand the surgical procedure or the risks involved. What should the nurse do?

    _____

    _____

    d. This nurse is normally assigned to a pediatric unit but was "floated" to Mr. Leonard's unit for the day. The nurse feels unfamiliar with the equipment and medications used with the clients on this unit. What is her responsibility?

    _____

    _____

    e. Could the nurse be held liable if Mr. Leonard suffers as a result of improper nursing care? How might personal malpractice or liability insurance help the nurse in this situation?

    _____

    _____

Self-Assessment Questions

Circle the letter that corresponds to the best answer for each question.

1. A nurse fails to verify a questionable order with the physician, resulting in harm to the client. This is an example of
   a. battery.
   b. negligence.
   c. malpractice.
   d. misdemeanor.

2. A client who resides in a facility that receives Medicare funding must
   a. forgo life-prolonging procedures.
   b. complete a living will document.
   c. initiate a durable power of attorney for health care.
   d. have the opportunity to complete an advance directive.

3. An incident or variance report is most useful in an institution to help
   a. clarify in the client's chart what happened in an incident.
   b. identify problem areas for possible lawsuits.
   c. prevent a lawsuit from being initiated.
   d. document poor professional activities.

4. A nurse is asked by a neighbor to look at her child who is ill. In this situation, the nurse would be
   a. liable for any harm caused by misdiagnosis or treatment.
   b. protected by his/her employer's liability policy.
   c. protected by the Good Samaritan Act.
   d. violating the nursing practice act.

5. The first priority for the nurse who suspects a colleague is using habit-forming drugs is to
   a. determine what laws may have been broken.
   b. document any incidences and report to a supervisor.
   c. report the colleague to the State Board of Nursing.
   d. confront the colleague with any suspicions.

Ethical Responsibilities

Key Terms

Match the following terms with their correct definitions.

___ 1. Active Euthanasia

    a. Individual's collection of inner beliefs that guides the way the person acts and helps determine the choices the person makes.

___ 2. Assisted Suicide

___ 3. Autonomy

    b. Application of general ethical principles to health care.

    c. Process of thinking through what one ought to do in an orderly, systematic manner based on principles.

___ 4. Beneficence

    d. Principles that influence the development of beliefs and attitudes.

___ 5. Bioethics

    e. Calling attention to unethical, illegal, or incompetent actions of others.

___ 6. Categorical Imperative

    f. Situation wherein there is a conflict between two or more ethical principles.

___ 7. Client Advocate

    g. Ethical theory that states that the value of a situation is determined by its consequences.

___ 8. Deontology

    h. Concept that states that one should act only if the action is based on a principle that is universal.

___ 9. Ethical Dilemma

    i. Process of taking deliberate action that will hasten a client's death.

___10. Ethical Principle

    j. Branch of philosophy concerned with determining right from wrong on the basis of a body of knowledge.

___11. Ethical Reasoning

    k. Ethical principle based on the concept of fairness extended to each individual.

___12. Ethics

    l. Person who speaks up for or acts on behalf of the client.

___13. Euthanasia

    m. Situation wherein another person provides a client with the means to end his own life.

___14. Fidelity

    n. Ethical principle based on the duty to promote good and prevent harm.

___15. Justice

    o. Process of analyzing one's own values to better understand those things that are truly important.

___16. Material Principle of Justice   p. Ethical principle that states that an act must result in the greatest degree of good for the greatest number of people involved in a given situation.

___17. Nonmaleficence   q. Ethical principle based on the individual's right to choose and the individual's ability to act on that choice.

___18. Passive Euthanasia   r. Ethical theory that considers the intrinsic significance of an act as the criterion for determination of good.

___19. Teleology   s. Ethical principle based on truthfulness (neither lying nor deceiving others).

___20. Utility   t. Widely accepted code, generally based on the humane aspects of society, that directs or governs actions.

___21. Value System   u. Intentional action or lack of action that causes the merciful death of someone suffering from a terminal illness or incurable condition; derived from the Greek word *euthanatos,* which means "good or gentle death."

___22. Values   v. Rationale for determining those times when there can be unequal allocation of scarce resources.

___23. Values Clarification   w. Process of cooperating with the client's dying process.

___24. Veracity   x. Ethical concept based on faithfulness and keeping promises.

___25. Whistleblowing   y. Ethical principle based on the obligation to cause no harm to others.

Abbreviation Review

Write the definition of the following abbreviations and acronyms.

1. AHA _____
2. ANA _____
3. ICN _____
4. LP/VN _____
5. NFL _____
6. VA _____

Exercises and Activities

1. Why do ethical dilemmas occur in health care?

   _____
   _____
   _____
   _____

a. Write your values or beliefs about each of the following issues.

Passive euthanasia: _____

_____

Active euthanasia: _____

_____

Assisted suicide: _____

_____

Refusal of treatment: _____

_____

Organ donation: _____

_____

b. How is the process of values clarification helpful to you?

_____

_____

2. Differentiate between each of the following terms:

Ethics vs. values

_____

_____

Ethical vs. legal

_____

_____

Nonmaleficence vs. negligence

_____

_____

Teleology vs. deontology

_____

_____

3. Complete each of the following statements:

a. Understanding ethical principles is important for the nurse because _____

_____

b. The nurse bases the care of clients on ethical behavior because _____

_____

c. The Code for Licensed Practical/Vocational Nurses is important because _____

_____

  d. If the nurse is faced with an ethical dilemma, the nurse should _____

  _____

4. Mrs. Nuñez gave birth to her fourth child 10 months ago. She received no prenatal care. The baby was diagnosed at birth with a serious genetic disorder that causes severe retardation, facial and skull abnormalities, and heart defects. Survival past a few months of age is rare. Mrs. Nuñez had originally been advised to withhold feedings and allow the infant to die. Instead, she chose to feed and care for her child at home in addition to her other children. Since then, however, Mrs. Nuñez has repeatedly brought the child back to the hospital for medical treatment, at great expense to the hospital. Members of the health care team have asked Mrs. Nuñez to meet with them to discuss her child's medical issues.

  a. For this situation, what are the ethical issues involved?

  _____

  _____

  b. In what way are each of the following ethical principles involved?

  Autonomy: _____

  _____

  Nonmaleficence: _____

  _____

  Justice: _____

  _____

  Veracity: _____

  _____

  c. What would be the consequences of providing or withholding care?

  _____

  _____

  d. Who should represent the interests of the child in this situation?

  _____

  e. Should the costs of providing care be a factor in any decisions?

  _____

  _____

  f. What is the nurse's role in this process?

  _____

  _____

Self-Assessment Questions

Circle the letter that corresponds to the best answer for each question.

1. The ethical foundation of the nurse-client relationship is the
   a. duty to promote good and prevent harm.
   b. principle of nonmaleficence.
   c. Patient's Bill of Rights.
   d. concept of fidelity.

2. The principle that an act must result in the greatest degree of good for the greatest number of people involved in a given situation is called
   a. utility.
   b. beneficence.
   c. client advocacy.
   d. situational theory.

3. The Patient's Bill of Rights is most useful to
   a. guide health care workers in treatment decisions.
   b. outline clients' responsibilities and ways they will be treated in the hospital.
   c. be a legally binding contract between health care workers and clients.
   d. provide a framework for ethical dilemmas.

4. If you are caring for a client whose value system conflicts with your own, you should first attempt to
   a. be aware of your own values.
   b. ask the client to clarify his/her values.
   c. engage in a meaningful dialogue with the client.
   d. determine which nursing actions you are willing to do.

5. An ethical dilemma in the health care setting is best resolved when the nurse
   a. asks the physician what to do.
   b. refers the issue to an ethics committee.
   c. refers to procedure manuals.
   d. uses ethical reasoning.

6. The first step in ethical decision making is to
   a. select a course of action.
   b. determine the claims of each party.
   c. identify who should make the decision.
   d. consider the likely consequences of actions.

Communication

Key Terms

Match the following terms with their correct definitions.

___ 1. Active Listening

___ 2. Aphasia

___ 3. Communication

___ 4. Congruent

___ 5. Dysarthria

___ 6. Dysphasia

___ 7. Empathy

___ 8. Feedback

___ 9. Hearing

___10. Listening

___11. Nonverbal Communication

___12. Proxemics

___13. Rapport

___14. Telemedicine

___15. Therapeutic Communication

___16. Verbal Communication

a. Communication that is purposeful and goal directed, creating a beneficial outcome for the client.

b. Sending a message without words; sometimes called body language.

c. Difficult and defective speech due to a dysfunction of the muscles used for speech.

d. Response from the receiver of a message so that the sender can verify the message.

e. Process of hearing spoken words and noting nonverbal behaviors.

f. Use of communications technology to transmit health information from one location to another.

g. Using words, either spoken or written, to send a message.

h. Interpreting the sounds heard and attaching meaning to them.

i. Relationship of mutual trust and understanding.

j. Impairment of speech resulting from damage to the speech center in the brain.

k. The sending and receiving of a message.

l. Study of the space between people and its effect on interpersonal behavior.

m. Act or power of receiving sounds.

n. Inability to communicate, the result of a brain lesion.

o. Agreement between two things.

p. Capacity to understand another person's feelings or perception of a situation.

Abbreviation Review

Write the definition of the following abbreviations and acronyms.

1. CPR _____
2. HIV _____
3. IOM _____
4. LP/VN _____
5. RN _____
6. WPM _____

Exercises and Activities

1. Look at each of these photographs and describe what types of nonverbal communication are present.

    a. What nonverbal communication does this nurse convey?

    _____
    _____
    _____
    _____
    _____
    _____
    _____
    _____
    _____
    _____
    _____
    _____

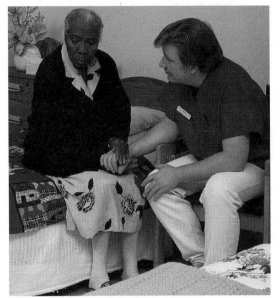

    b. What nonverbal communication do you observe in this client?

    _____
    _____
    _____
    _____
    _____
    _____
    _____
    _____
    _____
    _____
    _____

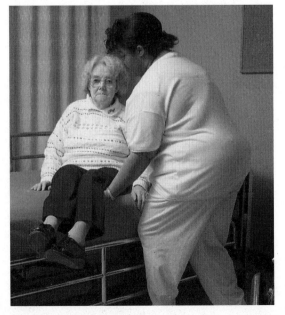

2. If you were having a conversation with a client right now, how might each of the following factors influence your communication style?

   a. Your age: _____

   _____

   b. Your education: _____

   _____

   c. Your emotions: _____

   _____

   d. Your culture: _____

   _____

   e. Your attention: _____

   _____

   f. Your surroundings: _____

   _____

3. For each of the following statements, give the communication technique being demonstrated. Does it have a positive or a negative effect? If it is negative, rewrite it in a way that might be therapeutic.

Nurse's Statement	Technique or Barrier Demonstrated	Rewrite if Necessary
a. "Tell me about your surgery last month."		
b. "You know the rules about visitors. They'll have to leave."		
c. "Well, I don't believe you should be doing that in your condition."		
d. "You look uncomfortable. Do you need more pain medication?"		
e. "Earlier you talked about feeling light-headed. Tell me more about that."		
f. "Every cloud has a silver lining."		

Nurse's Statement	*Technique or Barrier Demonstrated*	*Rewrite if Necessary*
g. "Under the circumstances, it was the only thing you could do."		
h. "What did you learn in the class this morning?"		

4. Mr. Singh is a 45-year-old client recently diagnosed with lung cancer. He is facing surgery tomorrow and appears very worried. At home, his wife is caring for their two children, ages 11 and 14. When you enter his room at the start of your shift, he is sitting quietly in bed and doesn't seem to hear you.

   a. What behaviors or attitudes might help you to communicate with Mr. Singh in a caring manner?

   _____

   _____

   b. How could you begin a conversation with him using one or more of the therapeutic communication techniques?

   _____

   _____

   c. How could you use silence in this situation?

   _____

   _____

Self-Assessment Questions

Circle the letter that corresponds to the best answer for each question.

1. The nurse caring for a client states, "A minute ago, you said you were sleeping poorly at night. Could you tell me more about that?" This is an example of
    a. focusing.
    b. restating.
    c. reflecting.
    d. paraphrasing.

2. The nurse practicing therapeutic communication will avoid
    a. silence.
    b. giving advice.
    c. using gestures.
    d. procedural touch.

3. The goals of therapeutic communication include
   a. self-disclosure, validation, and empathy.
   b. obtaining information, developing trust, and showing caring.
   c. active listening, data gathering, and developing a communication style.
   d. offering assistance, showing acceptance, and reducing communication blocks.

4. Imposing a personal set of values while caring for a client is a barrier to communication that is called
   a. validating.
   b. giving advice.
   c. value sharing.
   d. judgmental response.

5. To communicate with a client with dysphasia, the nurse will remember to
   a. speak normally.
   b. ask a family member to assist.
   c. touch the client's arm before speaking.
   d. use slightly exaggerated word formation.

6. During a conversation, a client reveals to you that she may be in an abusive relationship. As the nurse you realize that
   a. you can demonstrate caring by encouraging the client to share her fears.
   b. nurse-client communication is privileged and should be kept confidential.
   c. a client care conference will help determine what steps the client should take.
   d. you have a responsibilty to share the information with health care team members.

Cultural Diversity and Nursing

Key Terms

Match the following terms with their correct definitions.

____ 1. Acculturation

____ 2. Agnostic

____ 3. Atheist

____ 4. Cultural Assimilation

____ 5. Cultural Diversity

____ 6. Culture

____ 7. Dominant Culture

____ 8. Ethnicity

____ 9. Ethnocentrism

____10. Minority Group

____11. Oppression

____12. Race

a. Opposing forces that, when in balance, yield health.

b. Group of ministers, priests, rabbis, nuns, or laypersons who are able to meet clients' spiritual needs in the health care setting.

c. Cultural group's perception of itself or a group identity.

d. Process of learning norms, beliefs, and behavioral expectations of a group.

e. Process whereby individuals from a minority group are absorbed by the dominant culture and take on the characteristics of the dominant culture.

f. Dynamic and integrated structures of knowledge, beliefs, behaviors, ideas, attitudes, values, habits, customs, languages, symbols, rituals, ceremonies, and practices that are unique to a particular group of people.

g. Assumption of cultural superiority and an inability to accept other cultures' ways of organizing reality.

h. Condition wherein the rules, modes, and ideals of one group are imposed on another group.

i. Recognition of spiritual needs and the assistance given toward meeting those needs.

j. Individual who believes that the existence of God cannot be proved or disproved.

k. Differences among people that result from racial, ethnic, and cultural variables.

l. Group of people that constitute less than a numerical majority of the population and who, because of their cultural, racial, ethnic, religious, or other characteristics, are often labeled and treated differently from others in the society.

___13. Religious Support System

m. Individual's desire to find meaning and purpose in life, pain, and death.

___14. Spiritual Care

n. Individual who does not believe in God or any other deity.

___15. Spiritual Needs

o. Group whose values prevail within a society.

___16. Stereotyping

p. Grouping of people based on biological similarities such as physical characteristics.

___17. Yin and Yang

q. Belief that all people within the same racial, ethnic, or cultural group act alike and share the same beliefs and attitudes.

Abbreviation Review

Write the definition of the following acronym.

1. WHO _____

Exercises and Activities

1. How do the terms *ethnicity* and *race* differ?

   _____
   _____
   _____

   a. How would you explain the term *cultural diversity* to another student?

   _____
   _____
   _____

   b. In what ways does cultural diversity of health care workers, clients, and community populations affect you and your clients in today's health care settings?

   _____
   _____
   _____
   _____

2. Briefly describe your own cultural background and then complete the Cultural Assessment Interview Guide.

   _____
   _____
   _____
   _____
   _____

Cultural Assessment Interview Guide

Name: _____

Nickname or other names or special meaning attributed to your name: _____

Primary language:

      When speaking _____

      When writing _____

Date of birth: _____

Place of birth: _____

Educational level or specialized training: _____

To which ethnic group do you belong? _____

To what extent do you identify with your cultural group? _____

Who is the spokesperson for your family? _____

Describe some of the customs or beliefs that you have about the following:

      Health _____

      Life _____

      Illness _____

      Death _____

How do you best learn information?

    ☐ Reading

    ☐ Having someone explain verbally

    ☐ Having someone demonstrate

Describe some of your family's dietary habits and your personal food preferences: _____

_____

Are there any foods forbidden from your diet for religious or cultural reasons? _____

_____

Describe your religious affiliation: _____

What role do your religious beliefs and practices play in your life during times of good health and bad health? _____

_____

On whom do you rely on for health care services or healing, and to what type of cultural health practices have you been exposed? _____

_____

Are there any sanctions or restrictions in your culture about which the person taking care of you should know? _____

_____

Describe your current living arrangements: _____

How do members of your family communicate with each other? _____

Describe your strengths: _____

Who /what is your primary source of information about your health? _____

Is there anything else that is important about your cultural beliefs that you want to tell me? _____

From Fundamentals of Nursing: Standards & Practice, *by S. DeLaune and P. Ladner, 1998, Albany, NY: Delmar.*
Copyright 1998 by Delmar.

a. Choose two cultural groups different from your own. Compare their beliefs or customs for the following topics.

Cultural Group:_____   Cultural Group:_____

Family structure
Time orientation
Religion
What causes disease
Who provides health care
Special healing practices

b. How might each of the following affect health care practices?

Religious beliefs: _____

_____

Family structure: _____

_____

Time orientation: _____

_____

Nutritional preferences: _____

_____

3. In which cultural or religious group would you find each of the following beliefs or health practices?

_____ Cupping may be used to draw out evil or illness.
_____ A talisman worn around the wrist or neck wards off disease.
_____ A healing ritual called the Blessingway ceremony may be performed.
_____ Traditional healers include the curandero and yerbero.
_____ Prayers to Allah may be offered five times a day.
_____ Traditional healers include the shaman.
_____ Illness can be eliminated through prayer and spiritual understanding.
_____ Male circumcision is a religious custom performed 8 days after birth.
_____ Blood and blood products are usually refused.
_____ A special undergarment may be worn that symbolizes dedication to God.

a. Describe how you might feel about caring for each of the following clients.

A client who relies on "folk remedies" and healers: _____

_____

A client who responds to pain in a different way than you: _____

_____

A client who is using healing rituals and ceremonies: _____

_____

b. In what ways does each of the following religions support the spiritual needs of an ill client?

Christian Science: _____

_____

Judaism: _____

_____

Islam: _____

_____

Protestant: _____

_____

Roman Catholic _____

_____

4. You are assigned to care for Mrs. El Haddad, a 68-year-old client who has been admitted to your hospital for congestive heart failure. She and her husband have been in the United States for 2 months to visit their son and had planned on returning home before Mrs. El Haddad became ill. As you enter her room to do a physical assessment, you note that she is wearing traditional clothing with only her face and hands exposed, rather than a hospital gown. Her husband, who speaks limited English, sits next to her. Mrs. El Haddad appears anxious and uncomfortable but doesn't respond to your questions about pain. You want to help your client but are unfamiliar with her culture and religion.

a. In what ways can health care givers support Mrs. El Haddad's religious beliefs while she is hospitalized?

_____

_____

_____

b. List two nursing diagnoses with cultural implications that might be appropriate for your client.

(1) _____

(2) _____

c. How can members of her family assist you in providing culturally sensitive nursing care?

_____

_____

d. If you are caring for a client of a cultural or religious group with which you are unfamiliar, how could you determine the special needs or sources of support for your client?

_____

_____

_____

Self-Assessment Questions

Circle the letter that corresponds to the best answer for each question.

1. The first priority for the nurse providing culturally sensitive care is to
    a. accommodate differences when possible.
    b. identify the client's cultural/religious group.
    c. examine one's own culture and personal beliefs.
    d. listen for cues in the client's conversation about ethnic beliefs.

2. A time orientation to the past may be demonstrated by which of the following cultural groups?
    a. Asian American
    b. Native American
    c. African American
    d. Hispanic American

3. The process of learning the norms, beliefs, and behaviors of a culture is referred to as
    a. socialization.
    b. acculturation.
    c. ethnocentrism.
    d. cultural assimilation.

4. The nurse is caring for an Asian American client who refuses ice water and the cold foods served for her meal. The nurse recognizes that because of the client's cultural background, her refusal is most likely due to her
    a. attempt to cleanse her body of unhealthy organisms.
    b. acceptance of a supernatural cause for disease.
    c. belief in a yin and yang etiology of disease.
    d. preference for her own family's foods.

5. Which of the following statements is true concerning cultural influence on health care?
    a. All cultures value health and good medical practice.
    b. Response to health and illness varies according to cultural origin.
    c. Clients from all cultures respond positively to the nurse's caring touch.
    d. Knowing a client's cultural identity allows the nurse to make certain assumptions.

Wellness Concepts

Key Terms

Match the following terms with their correct definitions.

___ 1. Health

___ 2. Prevention

___ 3. Primary Prevention

___ 4. Secondary Prevention

___ 5. Tertiary Prevention

___ 6. Wellness

a. Early detection, diagnosis, screening, and intervention, generally before symptoms appear, to reduce the consequences of a health problem.

b. State of optimal health wherein an individual moves toward integration of human functioning, maximizes human potential, takes responsibility for health, and has greater self-awareness and self-satisfaction.

c. According to the World Health Organization, the state of complete physical, mental, and social well-being, not merely the absence of disease or infirmity.

d. Hindering, obstructing, or thwarting a disease or illness.

e. Treatment of an illness or disease after symptoms have appeared so as to prevent further progression.

f. All practices designed to keep health problems from developing.

Abbreviation Review

Write the definition of the following abbreviations and acronyms.

1. AIDS _____

2. CDC _____

3. ECG _____

4. EKG _____

5. Hgb _____

6. HIV _____

7. LDL _____

8. Pap _____

9. RBC _____

10. SPF _____

11. USDHHS _____

12. WHO _____

Exercises and Activities

1. Write your own definition of wellness as you believe it applies to you. Include behaviors in each of the seven areas of wellness: emotional, mental, intellectual, vocational, social, spiritual, and physical wellness.

   _____

   _____

   _____

   _____

   _____

   _____

   a. Choose three of the areas of wellness and describe what you could do to promote wellness for yourself in each of those areas.

      (1) _____

      (2) _____

      (3) _____

   b. Describe your concept of wellness as it might apply to an elderly client.

      _____

      _____

      _____

2. List three overall goals for the Healthy People 2000 objective.

   (1) _____

   (2) _____

   (3) _____

3. Review Table 7-1 in your text. Look at the objectives for physical activity and fitness, nutrition, and AIDS/HIV infection. Briefly describe each objective and state whether the objective met the Year 2000 target. If the target was not met, give a possible reason.

   Physical Activity and Fitness _____

   _____

   Nutrition _____

   _____

   AIDS/HIV infection _____

   _____

4. In what ways can nurses be involved in helping to achieve the goals of Healthy People 2010?

   _____

   _____

   _____

5. Why is the individual at the center of the health care team?

_____

_____

_____

6. List the four factors affecting health. Describe the role each factor plays in determining the health of an individual.

(1) _____

(2) _____

(3) _____

(4) _____

7. Define each type of prevention and give two examples.

	Definition	*Examples*
Primary		(1) (2)
Secondary		(1) (2)
Tertiary		(1) (2)

8. Nicole Taylor is a 20-year-old college student who is studying computer programming. Although she finds her courses interesting, she is becoming increasingly stressed about her class load and grades. Struggling to maintain a passing average, she has started smoking again, after having quit 6 months ago. She has also regained several pounds that she had previously lost through diet and exercise. To pay for classes, Nicole works 25 hours a week at a restaurant. Her boyfriend, with whom she is sexually active, tries to be supportive. Because of her current schedule she has little time for exercise, and she knows she shouldn't be smoking, but doesn't think she can quit again.

a. What health problems might Nicole encounter if she continues with her present lifestyle?

_____

_____

b. What changes would be most helpful to Nicole at this time?

_____

_____

c. Recommend three methods of stress reduction for Nicole to try.

_____

_____

_____

  d. At Nicole's age, what routine exams would you suggest she have?

  _____

  _____

  e. After reviewing a genogram with information regarding Nicole's family, you determine
      that she is at increased risk for osteoporosis. What steps could you recommend to Nicole
      that might prevent or reduce her risk for this disease?

  _____

  _____

Self-Assessment Questions

Circle the letter that corresponds to the best answer for each question.

1. Which of the following areas has the most factors affecting health and wellness?
    a. Genetics and human biology
    b. Environmental influences
    c. Personal behavior
    d. Health care

2. Monthly breast self-examination is an example of which of the following?
    a. Primary prevention
    b. Secondary prevention
    c. Tertiary prevention
    d. Early intervention

3. A major goal of Healthy People 2000/2010 is to
    a. increase access to preventive services.
    b. provide more health care workers.
    c. establish health care guidelines.
    d. identify concepts of wellness.

4. An important part of tertiary prevention is
    a. screening.
    b. rehabilitation.
    c. health promotion.
    d. consumer awareness.

5. A client who is experiencing excessive stress is at risk for accidents, heart disease, and
    a. stroke.
    b. cancer.
    c. diabetes.
    d. atherosclerosis.

Alternative/Complementary Therapies

Key Terms

Match the following terms with their correct definitions.

___ 1. Acupressure

___ 2. Acupuncture

___ 3. Alternative Therapies

___ 4. Antioxidant

___ 5. Aromatherapy

___ 6. Biofeedback

___ 7. Bodymind

___ 8. Centering

___ 9. Complementary Therapies

___ 10. Curing

___ 11. Energetic-Touch Therapies

___ 12. Free Radicals

___ 13. Healing

a. Ridding of disease.

b. Altered state of consciousness or awareness resembling sleep and during which a person is more receptive to suggestion.

c. Folk healer-priest who uses natural and supernatural forces to help others.

d. Therapies used instead of conventional or mainstream medical practices.

e. Nonnutritive, physiologically active compounds present in plants in very small amounts; store nutrients and provide structure, aroma, flavor, and color.

f. Technique of releasing blocked energy within an individual when specific points (Tsubas) along the meridians are pressed or massaged by the practitioner's fingers, thumbs, and heel of the hands.

g. Measurement of physiological responses that yields information about the relationship between the mind and body and helps clients learn the way to manipulate these responses through mental activity.

h. Energy-based therapeutic modality that alters the energy fields through the use of touch, thereby affecting physical, mental, emotional, and spiritual health.

i. Quieting of the mind by focusing the attention.

j. Relaxation technique of using the imagination to visualize a pleasant, soothing image.

k. Therapies used in conjunction with conventional medical therapies.

l. A means by which healing can be achieved, performed, or enhanced.

m. Therapeutic use of concentrated essences or essential oils that have been extracted from plants and flowers.

___14. Healing Touch

n. Technique of application of heat and needles to various points on the body to alter the energy flow.

___15. Hypnosis

o. Inseparable connection and operation of thoughts, feelings, and physiological functions.

___16. Imagery

p. Amino acids produced in the brain and other sites in the body that act as chemical communicators.

___17. Instrument of Healing

q. Study of the complex relationship among the cognitive, affective, and physical aspects of humans.

___18. Meditation

r. Application of pressure and motion by the hands with the intent of improving the recipient's well-being.

___19. Neuropeptides

s. Process of bringing oneself to an inward focus of serenity, done before beginning an energetic-touch therapy treatment.

___20. Neurotransmitters

t. Unstable molecules that alter genetic codes and trigger the development of cancer growth in cells.

___21. Phytochemicals

u. A technique of assessing alterations in a person's energy fields and using the hands to direct energy to achieve a balanced state.

___22. Psychoneuroimmunology

v. Chemical substances produced by the body that facilitate nerve-impulse transmission.

___23. Shaman

w. Means of perceiving or experiencing through tactile sensation.

___24. Shamanism

x. Practice of entering altered states of consciousness with the intent of helping others.

___25. Therapeutic Massage

y. Substance that prevents or inhibits oxidation, a chemical process wherein a substance is joined to oxygen.

___26. Therapeutic Touch

z. Techniques of using the hands to direct or redirect the flow of the body's energy fields and thus enhance balance within those fields.

___27. Touch

aa. Process that activates the individual's recovery forces from within.

Abbreviation Review

Write the definition of the following acronyms.

1. AHNA _____

2. FDA _____

3. LDL _____

4. NCCAM _____

5. OAM _____

6. PMR _____

7. PNI _____

Exercises and Activities

1. How would you describe nursing as holistic?

   _____

   _____

   _____

   a. How would you explain the concept of the bodymind to another student?

      _____

      _____

2. For each of the following cultures, briefly describe their health perception and give examples of current therapies based on those beliefs.

Culture	Health Perception	Current Therapies
Greek culture		
Far East		
China		
India		
Shamanism		

3. Differentiate among the following terms: therapeutic massage; therapeutic touch; healing touch.

   _____

   _____

   _____

   a. Briefly describe the five phases of therapeutic touch.

      (1) _____

      (2) _____

      (3) _____

      (4) _____

      (5) _____

4. List two primary benefits of each of the following alternative/complementary therapies and the types of conditions they may help.

Therapy		Primary Benefits	Types of Conditions
Guided imagery	(1)		
	(2)		
Biofeedback	(1)		
	(2)		
Yoga	(1)		
	(2)		
Shiatsu/acupressure	(1)		
	(2)		

   a. Using Table 8-4, Medicinal Value of Herbs, name two herbs a holistic practitioner might use for each of these conditions.

   Healing a wound: _____

   Mild depression: _____

   Headache: _____

   Common cold/sinus congestion: _____

   b. Why are nurses cautioned against the casual use of herbal therapy?

   _____

   _____

5. You have been working as an LP/VN at a long-term care facility since your graduation 6 months ago. The facility is pleasant, nicely decorated, and home to sixty-four residents. You particularly enjoy caring for Mr. Reiner, whose daughter and granddaughter visit twice a week. On her most recent visit, the daughter mentions how much her father enjoyed his dog at home, a black Labrador retriever. She asks if this facility ever thought about having a pet therapy program. Apparently, she tells you, many long-term care facilities are using pet therapy with very good results. You mention it to the supervising nurse, who asks you to evaluate the idea.

   a. In what ways might a pet therapy program benefit the clients in this facility?

   _____

   _____

   b. What issues would you need to consider?

   _____

   _____

   _____

   c. What other types of complementary therapies might you consider for this facility?

   _____

   _____

d. You ask Mr. Reiner if he would like to join an exercise group that meets 3 times a week in the social activities room. What benefits would a regular exercise group have for Mr. Reiner and other residents?

_____

_____

_____

Self-Assessment Questions

Circle the letter that corresponds to the best answer for each question.

1. The use of complementary/alternative therapies is increasing because most are
   a. noninvasive and less expensive.
   b. covered by insurance.
   c. easy to learn at home.
   d. spiritual in nature.

2. Because nursing deals with physiological, psychological, sociological, intellectual, and spiritual aspects of the individual, nursing can be described as
   a. comprehensive.
   b. complemental.
   c. humanistic.
   d. holistic.

3. The nurse explains that the benefits of meditation for the client include
   a. decreased oxygen consumption and blood pressure.
   b. enhanced stamina, agility, and balance.
   c. restoration of sensation and function.
   d. increased heart rate and lactic acid.

4. Chiropractic therapy is an example of which category of alternative/complementary intervention?
   a. Energetic touch
   b. Body movement
   c. Mind/body therapy
   d. None of the above

5. The first phase for the nurse preparing to use therapeutic touch with a client is called
   a. reflection.
   b. assessment.
   c. evaluation.
   d. centering.

6. Reflexology is an alternative/complementary therapy based on the
   a. shamanistic tradition.
   b. human energy fields.
   c. ancient healing arts.
   d. Ayurvedic system.

7. The nurse understands that massage therapy
    a. is also called therapeutic touch.
    b. is useful with clients from all cultural backgrounds.
    c. may be contraindicated in hypertension and diabetes.
    d. is a treatment modality specified in the nursing practice act.

Loss, Grief, and Death

Key Terms

Match the following terms with their correct definitions.

___ 1. Algor Mortis

___ 2. Anticipatory Grief

___ 3. Autopsy

___ 4. Bereavement

___ 5. Breakthrough Pain

___ 6. Cheyne-Stokes Respirations

___ 7. Complicated Grief

___ 8. Death Rattle

___ 9. Disenfranchised Grief

___10. Dysfunctional Grief

___11. Grief

___12. Grief Work

___13. Health Care Surrogate Law

a. Breathing characterized by periods of apnea alternating with periods of dyspnea.

b. Persistent pattern of intense grief that does not result in reconciliation of feelings.

c. Process whereby the bereaved experiences freedom from attachment to the deceased, becomes reoriented to the environment where the deceased is no longer present, and establishes new relationships.

d. Form of reminiscence wherein a client attempts either to come to terms with conflict or to gain meaning from life and die peacefully.

e. Loss that occurs as a result of moving from one developmental stage to another.

f. Period of grief following the death of a loved one.

g. Care given immediately after death before the body is moved to the mortuary.

h. Covering for the body after death.

i. Decrease in body temperature after death, resulting in lack of skin elasticity.

j. Grief associated with traumatic death such as death by homicide, violence, or accident; survivors suffer emotions of greater intensity than those associated with normal grief.

k. Bluish purple discoloration of the skin, usually at pressure points, that is a by-product of red blood cell destruction.

l. Funeral home.

m. Occurrence of grief work before an expected loss actually occurs.

____14. Hospice

n. Care that relieves symptoms, such as pain, but does not alter the course of disease.

____15. Life Review

o. Stiffening of the body that occurs 2 to 4 hours after death as a result of contraction of skeletal and smooth muscles.

____16. Liver Mortis

p. Sudden, acute, temporary pain that is usually precipitated by a treatment, a procedure, or unusual activity of the client.

____17. Loss

q. "Grief that is not openly acknowledged, socially sanctioned, or publicly shared" (Doka, Rushton, & Thorstenson [1994]).

____18. Maturational Loss

r. Law enacted by some states that provides a legal means for decision making in the absence of advance directives.

____19. Mortuary

s. Support measures implemented to restore consciousness and life.

____20. Mourning

t. Grief reaction that normally follows a significant loss.

____21. Palliative Care

u. Any situation, either actual, potential, or perceived, wherein a valued object or person is changed or is no longer accessible to the individual.

____22. Post-Mortem Care

v. Examination of a body after death by a pathologist to determine cause of death.

____23. Resuscitation

w. Breathing sound in the period preceding death caused by a collection of secretions in the larynx.

____24. Rigor Mortis

x. Care for the terminally ill founded on the concept of allowing individuals to die with dignity and surrounded by those who love them.

____25. Shroud

y. Loss that occurs in response to external events that are usually beyond the individual's control.

____26. Situational Loss

z. Period of time during which grief is expressed and resolution and integration of the loss occur.

____27. Uncomplicated Grief

aa. Series of intense physical and psychological responses that occurs following a loss; a normal, natural, necessary, and adaptive response to a loss.

Abbreviation Review

Write the definition of the following acronyms.

1. ANA _____

2. DNR _____

3. HMO _____

4. IM _____

5. MS _____

6. NANDA _____

7. OBRA _____

8. PSDA _____

9. PTSD _____

10. SIDS _____

Exercises and Activities

1. Why is mourning an important process to an individual who is experiencing a loss?

   _____

   _____

   _____

   a. Describe an individual's reactions to loss according to Engle.

      _____

      _____

   b. Briefly describe each of the following types of loss.

      External object: _____

      Familiar environment: _____

      Aspect of self: _____

      Significant other: _____

   c. Give two examples of loss for each developmental stage.

      Early adulthood   (1) _____

                                    (2) _____

      Middle adulthood   (1) _____

                                    (2) _____

      Late adulthood   (1) _____

                                    (2) _____

2. Choose one type of loss that you have experienced. Briefly describe the loss and any feelings of grief that may have accompanied it.

   _____

   _____

   _____

   a. Did your feelings of grief resolve? If so, how long did the process take?

      _____

      _____

   b. What actions or statements by others were most helpful?

      _____

      _____

c. Were any actions or statements not helpful?

_____

_____

3. Differentiate between dysfunctional and disenfranchised grief.

_____

_____

_____

a. Why might an abortion cause an individual to experience disenfranchised grief?

_____

_____

b. Why is the loss of a child considered one of the most difficult?

_____

_____

4. One of your clients today is Mrs. Negassi, a 25-year-old woman who is terminally ill with ovarian cancer, diagnosed shortly after the birth of her second child a few months ago. She had completed a round of chemotherapy that was extremely difficult for her, with little effect on the cancer. After much thought she has made the decision not to continue therapy. Her primary concern now is her husband and the welfare of her children. Mr. Negassi appears to be in denial at times, and at others is angry with her physician for not diagnosing the disease earlier. There are many issues he needs to face, including taking over the care of both children.

a. According to Kübler-Ross's stages of dying and death, what stage do you feel Mrs. Negassi is in?

_____

What stage is her husband in?

_____

b. How might anticipatory grief be helpful for her husband?

_____

How might it be a disadvantage?

_____

_____

c. What role could hospice play in helping the client and family cope with her impending death?

_____

_____

d. Mrs. Negassi and her husband have finally discussed her wishes concerning terminal care. What documents should she complete?

_____

_____

   e. As death becomes imminent, list four physiological changes that occur and signs or symptoms that accompany each.

     (1) _____

     (2) _____

     (3) _____

     (4) _____

   f. You find yourself having difficulty dealing with Mrs. Negassi's death as you had become fond of her and very involved in her care. What symptoms might indicate that you are in need of grief counseling? What actions might be helpful to deal with the loss?

_____

_____

_____

_____

Self-Assessment Questions

Circle the letter that corresponds to the best answer for each question.

1. Your client experienced the death of her spouse several months ago. She continues to talk about him and the death repeatedly and is having difficulty eating and sleeping. This client is experiencing
   a. absent grief.
   b. detachment.
   c. dysfunctional grief.
   d. loss of patterns of conduct.

2. The nurse is caring for a client with terminal cancer. Nursing interventions for this client that focus on relieving symptoms such as pain are called
   a. respite care.
   b. palliative care.
   c. adjuvant therapy.
   d. anticipatory support.

3. The widow of a client who died violently three months ago is now being seen in the clinic for sleep disturbance and chronic anxiety, and may be experiencing PTSD. To support this client through the grief process, she will first be encouraged to
   a. fully accept the loss.
   b. begin to renew relationships
   c. express intense feelings she may have.
   d. become involved in outside interests and activities.

4. The nurse understands that a client with a living will and durable power of attorney
   a. is required to sign the Patient Self-Determination form.
   b. relinquishes the right to make health care decisions.
   c. has a life-threatening disease or terminal illness.
   d. still needs a "do not resuscitate" medical order.

5. According to Kübler-Ross, the fifth and final stage of dying experienced by an individual is
   a. life review.
   b. resignation.
   c. acceptance.
   d. hopefulness.

Fluid, Electrolyte, and Acid–Base Balance

Key Terms

Match the following terms with their correct definitions.

___ 1. Acid

___ 2. Acidosis

___ 3. Alkalosis

___ 4. Anion

___ 5. Arterial Blood Gases (ABGs)

___ 6. Atom

___ 7. Base

___ 8. Buffer

___ 9. Cation

___10. Compound

___11. Crenation

___12. Decomposition

___13. Dehydration

___14. Dialysis

a. Decreased oxygen level in the blood.

b. Pressure that a fluid exerts against a membrane; also called filtration force.

c. Solution that has the same molecular concentration as does the cell; also called an isosmolar solution.

d. Substances combined in no specific way.

e. Measurement of levels of oxygen, carbon dioxide, pH, partial pressure of oxygen (PO_2 or PaO_2), partial pressure of carbon dioxide (PCO_2 or $PaCO_2$), saturation of oxygen (SaO_2), and bicarbonate (HCO_2) in arterial blood.

f. Substance that attempts to maintain pH range, or hydrogen ion concentration, in the presence of added acids or bases.

g. Condition wherein cells decrease in size, shrivel and wrinkle, and are no longer functional when in a hypertonic solution.

h. Condition wherein more water is lost from the body than is being replaced.

i. Seepage of fluid into the interstitial tissue as a result of accidental dislodgement of the IV needle from the vein.

j. Pressure exerted against the cell membrane by the water inside a cell.

k. Membrane that allows passage of only certain substances.

l. Normal resiliency of the skin.

m. Equilibrium (balance); consistency of body fluids.

n. Rupture of red blood cells due to osmosis.

___15. Diffusion

___16. Edema

___17. Electrolyte

___18. Element

___19. Extracellular Fluid

___20. Filtration

___21. Hemolysis

___22. Homeostasis

___23. Hydrostatic Pressure

___24. Hypertonic Solution

___25. Hypotonic Solution

___26. Hypoxemia

___27. Infiltration

___28. Interstitial Fluid

___29. Intracellular Fluid

___30. Intravascular Fluid

___31. Intravenous Therapy

___32. Ion

___33. Isotonic Solution

___34. Isotopes

___35. Matter

o. Administration of fluids, electrolytes, nutrients, or medications by the venous route.

p. Fluid in tissue spaces around each cell.

q. Measurement of the total concentration of dissolved particles (solutes) per kilogram of water.

r. Diffusion used to separate molecules out of a solution by passing them through a semipermeable membrane.

s. Substance that when dissociated produces ions that will combine with hydrogen ions.

t. Condition characterized by an excessive number of hydrogen ions in a solution.

u. In a solution, liquid, or gas, movement of molecules from an area of high molecular concentration to one of low molecular concentration.

v. Element or compound that, when dissolved in water or another solvent, dissociates (separates) into ions (electrically charged particles).

w. Fluid within the cells.

x. Atoms of the same element that have different atomic weights (i.e., different numbers of neutrons in the nucleus).

y. Product formed when an acid and a base react with each other.

z. Concentration of solutes per liter of cellular fluid.

aa. Anything that occupies space and possesses mass.

bb. Ion bearing a positive charge.

cc. Condition characterized by an excessive loss of hydrogen ions from a solution.

dd. Smallest unit of an element that still retains the properties of that element that cannot be altered by any chemical change.

ee. Detectable accumulation of increased interstitial fluid.

ff. Solution that has a lower molecular concentration than the cell; also called hypo-osmolar solution.

gg. Process of fluids and the substances dissolved in them being forced through the cell membrane by hydrostatic pressure.

hh. Diffusion from a region of higher concentration to a region of lower concentration.

ii. Joined with oxygen.

___36. Mixture

jj. Chemical reaction when two or more atoms, called reactants, bond and form a more complex molecular product.

___37. Molecule

kk. Fluid outside of the cells; includes interstitial, intravascular, synovial, cerebrospinal, and serous fluids; aqueous and vitreous humor; and endolymph and perilymph.

___38. Osmolality

ll. Fluid consisting of the plasma in the blood vessels and the lymph in the lymphatic system.

___39. Osmolarity

mm. Atoms of the same element that unite with each other.

___40. Osmosis

nn. Ability of a membrane to permit substances to pass through it.

___41. Osmotic Pressure

oo. Any substance that in a solution yields hydrogen ions bearing a positive charge.

___42. Oxidized

pp. Ion bearing a negative charge.

___43. Permeability

qq. Combination of atoms of two or more elements.

___44. Salt

rr. Chemical reaction wherein the bonding between atoms in a molecule is broken and simpler products are formed.

___45. Semipermeable Membrane

ss. Solution that has a higher molecular concentration than the cell; also called a hyperosmolar solution.

___46. Synthesis

tt. Basic substance of matter.

___47. Turgor

uu. Atom bearing an electrical charge.

Abbreviation Review

Write the meaning or definition of the following abbreviations, acronyms, and symbols.

1. ABG _____
2. ADH _____
3. ATP _____
4. BUN _____
5. Ca_+ _____
6. $CaCl_2$ _____
7. Cl^- _____
8. CO_2^- _____
9. COOH _____
10. D_5W _____
11. dL _____
12. ECF _____
13. H^+ _____
14. H_2CO_3 _____

15. H_2O _____

16. HCl _____

17. HCO_3^- _____

18. Hct _____

19. Hgb _____

20. I&O _____

21. ICF _____

22. K^+ _____

23. KCl _____

24. kg _____

25. L _____

26. lb _____

27. mEq _____

28. mg _____

29. Mg^{++} _____

30. MgCl _____

31. mL _____

32. mm Hg _____

33. MOM _____

34. mOsm/kg _____

35. Na^+ _____

36. Na_2HPO_4 _____

37. Na_2SO_4 _____

38. NaCl _____

39. NaH_2PO_4 _____

40. $NaHCO_3$ _____

41. $NaHPO_4$ _____

42. NaOH _____

43. NH_2 _____

44. O_2 _____

45. OH _____

46. PCO_2 ($PaCO_2$) _____

47. pH _____

48. PO_2 (PaO_2) _____

49. PO_4^{--} _____

50. SaO_2 _____

51. TPN _____

52. TPR _____

53. wt _____

Exercises and Activities

1. Complete the following statements:
   a. Understanding fluid and electrolyte balance is important for the nurse because

   _____

   _____

   b. Homeostasis can be described as

   _____

   _____

   c. The body tries to maintain homeostasis by

   _____

   _____

2. Use the following diagrams to describe the processes of osmosis and diffusion.

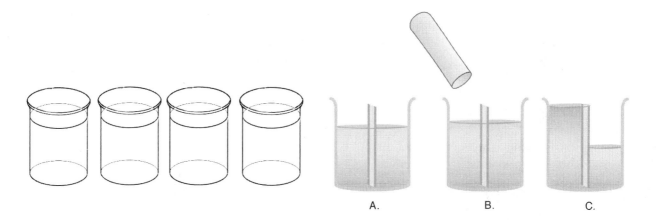

Draw and explain diffusion: Draw and explain osmosis:

   a. What is hemolysis and how does it occur?

   _____

   _____

    b. How does dialysis work?

    _____

    _____

3. Why is it important for the body to maintain the acid–base balance?

    _____

    _____

    _____

    a. How does each of the body's three main control systems regulate acid–base balance?

    The buffer systems: _____

    _____

    _____

    Respiratory regulation: _____

    _____

    _____

    Renal regulation: _____

    _____

    _____

    b. Which control system is fastest? _____

    Which control system is slowest? _____

4. List signs of a fluid imbalance that a nurse might observe on physical examination of a client.
   Fluid volume excess:

    (1) _____

    (2) _____

    (3) _____

    (4) _____

Fluid volume deficit:

    (1) _____

    (2) _____

    (3) _____

    (4) _____

    a. Why is dehydration a common and serious fluid imbalance in an individual?

    _____

    _____

    b. What are the primary nursing goals for a client with dehydration?

    _____

    _____

c. Explain why 0.9% NaCl could be used for fluid replacement.

_____

_____

d. What would you tell a client about the role that water plays in health?

_____

_____

5. Mr. Patel is a 29-year-old client who arrived at the hospital with multiple trauma following an automobile accident. Because of injury to his lungs, Mr. Patel is now acutely ill. On assessment, the nurse notes that Mr. Patel is showing signs of hypoxemia, including dyspnea, increased respiratory rate, and an increased heart rate. He has been restless since he was admitted, but now appears to be showing some confusion.

a. The nurse determines that Mr. Patel is exhibiting signs of which acid–base imbalance?

_____

_____

b. What changes in laboratory values would you anticipate?
pH _____
PCO^2 _____
HCO^3 _____

c. Why is a prompt and careful respiratory assessment important for this client?

_____

_____

d. List three actual or risk nursing diagnoses for Mr. Patel.
(1) _____
(2) _____
(3) _____

e. How does respiratory acidosis differ from metabolic acidosis?

_____

_____

Self-Assessment Questions

Circle the letter that corresponds to the best answer for each question.

1. The human body can tolerate only very slight changes in the
   a. fluid volume.
   b. metabolic rate.
   c. respiratory rate.
   d. blood pH value.

2. If the blood pH falls below 7.35, acidosis occurs, which may be characterized by a weak and irregular heartbeat, lower blood pressure, and
   a. a decrease in the LOC.
   b. a decreased respiratory rate.
   c. spasmodic muscle contractions.
   d. numbness and tingling in the extremities.

3. A client admitted with dehydration may exhibit signs and symptoms that include dry mucous membranes, decreased tearing, decreased urine output, and
   a. decreased pulse rate.
   b. lower blood pressure.
   c. jugular vein distention.
   d. taut, smooth, shiny, pale skin.

4. The hormones ADH, aldosterone, and renin are important to a client's health status because they
   a. maintain the fluid balance by encouraging the kidneys to retain water.
   b. maintain the acid-base balance by causing the excretion of sodium.
   c. stabilize the normal pH level as part of the buffer systems.
   d. bind with excess hydrogen ions in the blood.

5. A client tells the nurse that he has been taking a lot of antacid tablets and milk in an attempt to control heartburn. The nurse should be aware that this client may be at risk for
   a. gastric acidosis.
   b. metabolic acidosis.
   c. metabolic alkalosis.
   d. compensatory alkalosis.

6. The most common indicator in a client who has fluid volume deficit is
   a. thirst.
   b. weakness.
   c. decreased urination.
   d. increased skin turgor.

7. A client has been advised to take a calcium supplement. To increase her absorption of calcium from the gastrointestinal tract, the nurse explains to the client that she should also consume
   a. Vitamin C.
   b. Vitamin D.
   c. amino acids.
   d. sports drinks.

IV Therapy

Key Terms

Match the following terms with their correct definitions.

___ 1. Angiocatheter

a. Device made of a radiopaque silicone catheter and a plastic or stainless steel injection port with a self-sealing silicone-rubber septum.

___ 2. Butterfly Needle

b. Seepage of foreign substances into the interstitial tissue, causing swelling and discomfort at the IV site.

___ 3. Drug Incompatibility

c. Addition of an intravenous solution to infuse concurrently with another infusion.

___ 4. Flashback

d. Method of administering a large dose of medication in a relatively short time, usually 1 to 30 minutes.

___ 5. Flow Rate

e. Medication that causes blisters and tissue injury when it escapes into surrounding tissue.

___ 6. Hypervolemia

f. Increased circulating fluid volume.

___ 7. Implantable Port

g. Wing-tipped needle.

___ 8. Infiltration

h. Intracatheter with a metal stylet.

___ 9. Intracath

i. Plastic tube for insertion into a vein.

___10. Intravenous Therapy

j. Inflammation of a vein.

___11. IV Push (bolus)

k. Undesired chemical or physical reaction between a drug and a solution, between two drugs, or between a drug and the container or tubing.

___12. Phlebitis

l. Volume of fluid to infuse over a set period of time.

___13. Piggyback

m. Administration of fluids, electrolytes, nutrients, or medications by the venous route.

___14. Vesicant

n. Rushing of blood back into intravenous tubing when a negative pressure is created on the tubing.

Abbreviation Review

Write the meaning or definition of the following abbreviations, acronyms, and symbols.

1. CVC _____

2. D_5W _____

3. IV _____

4. IVPB _____

5. KVO _____

6. L _____

7. mL _____

8. PI _____

9. VAD _____

Exercises and Activities

1. List several reasons why a client might require continuous or intermittent IV therapy.

   _____

   _____

   _____

   a. Identify infection control practices that protect the client on IV therapy.

      _____

      _____

      _____

   b. What safety measures can help protect the nurse?

      _____

      _____

      _____

2. Your client is to begin IV therapy with 1000 cc D_5W to infuse over 12 hours. List all the items you will need to start the IV.

   _____

   _____

   _____

   a. State the principles that will guide you in selecting an appropriate IV site.

      _____

      _____

      _____

   b. What contraindications may exist for a particular site?

      (1) _____

      (2) _____

      (3) _____

      (4) _____

      (5) _____

c. Briefly describe the procedure for starting the IV.

_____

_____

_____

d. How many mL per hour will your client be receiving?_____ If the IV tubing has a drop factor of 15 drops/mL, the actual infusion rate will be _____ drops/min. What might be the advantage of using a volume controller or pump?

_____

_____

_____

e. After the IV has been started, what will you document?

_____

_____

_____

f. What routine assessment and documentation are required for a client on IV therapy?

_____

_____

_____

3. Why is it important to monitor for signs of phlebitis?

_____

_____

_____

a. List several signs and symptoms for a client with catheter sepsis.

(1) _____   (4) _____

(2) _____   (5) _____

(3) _____   (6) _____

b. If you are caring for an older client, what special precautions would be important?

_____

_____

_____

c. Describe nursing actions for the client experiencing a reaction to a blood product.

_____

_____

_____

4. Kim, a new nurse, has recently finished her orientation to a busy medical-surgical unit at the hospital near her home. She has just made rounds and is now preparing to give medications to several clients this morning. Kim notes that many of her clients are using IV therapy.

a. Her first client, Mr. Jenkins, is on continuous IV therapy. Kim notices that he needs one more bag of 1000 mL of NS, scheduled to infuse at a rate of 150 mL/hr. Since Kim is starting it at 0830, when will it finish? _____   At 1030, Mr. Jenkins' physician writes a new order to slow the IV infusion rate to 100 mL/hour. Now what time will this IV bag be finished? _____

b. In the next room, Kim will start the first of two antibiotics due at 9 A.M., IVPB, for Mrs. Johnson. Why will she check drug compatibility on the two medications?

_____

_____

_____

c. Before starting the first antibiotic, Kim assesses the IV site in Mrs. Johnson's right forearm. Mrs. Johnson tells her that the IV is starting to hurt a little. Kim recalls that the signs and symptoms of infiltration and phlebitis are:

_____

_____

_____

d. Kim has now determined that Mrs. Johnson has phlebitis, so she will:

_____

_____

_____

e. In the next room, Kim needs to reset the flow rate for an IV that is infusing in her client, Mr. Colvin. The new order is for 1000 mL of D_5/NS to infuse over 12 hours. She knows the infusion rate will be _____ mL/hour. Since Kim is not using an infusion pump, she will calculate the IV drip rate. The drop factor for this IV tubing is 10 drops/mL. Kim determines that the actual infusion rate is _____ drops/minute.

f. Depending on lab work this morning, Mrs. Henley, her last client, may need to have packed RBCs administered again today. Kim reviews the hospital's policy regarding blood transfusions. What items will Kim include in her initial assessment and preparation for Mrs. Henley to receive blood products?

_____

_____

_____

_____

_____

Self-Assessment Questions

Circle the letter that corresponds to the best answer for each question.

1. Which of the following statements is incorrect regarding the safety precautions used for IV therapy?
   a. Intracaths are changed every 3 days.
   b. IV solution bags that feel wet are discarded.
   c. Alcohol with Betadine is used for antiseptic cleansing.
   d. An IV filter reduces the risk of bacteremia and phlebitis.

2. A nurse is assessing the IV site on a client and notes the presence of swelling and cool, pale skin. The nurse understands that these are signs of
   a. phlebitis.
   b. infiltration.
   c. catheter sepsis.
   d. rapid IV infusion.

3. The nurse is preparing to administer IV fluids to a client. The physician's order is for 1000 mL to be infused over eight hours using IV tubing with a drop factor of 12 drops/mL. The nurse determines the actual infusion rate is approximately
   a. 125 cc/hour
   b. 21 drops/minute.
   c. 25 drops/minute.
   d. the same as if the drop factor was 10 drops/mL.

4. The nurse is administering an IVPB medication that is incompatible with the primary IV solution. Which of the following statements accurately describes the technique to administer the IVPB medication in this situation?
   a. Establish a new IV access via another peripheral vein.
   b. Back flush the secondary medication line with the primary solution.
   c. Use a volume-control set to run the IVPB medication at a slower rate than normal.
   d. Flush the primary line with NS before and after administering the IVPB medication.

5. Which of the following nursing activities would be performed first for the client who is receiving blood products?
   a. Take a baseline set of vital signs.
   b. Check to ensure the client has an 18-gauge or larger IV access.
   c. Verify the client's blood type and Rh with those of the blood product.
   d. Begin administration of the blood product within 30 minutes after receiving it.

Health Assessment

Key Terms

Match the following terms with their correct definitions.

___ 1. Adventitious Breath Sound

___ 2. Affect

___ 3. Auscultation

___ 4. Borborygmi

___ 5. Bradycardia

___ 6. Bradypnea

___ 7. Bronchial Sound

___ 8. Bronchovesicular Sound

___ 9. Crackle

___10. Cyanosis

___11. Dyspnea

___12. Eupnea

___13. Health History

___14. Hyperventilation

a. High-pitched, loud, rushing sounds produced by the movement of gas in the liquid contents of the intestine.

b. Physical examination technique that uses the sense of touch to assess texture, temperature, moisture, organ location and size, vibrations and pulsations, swelling, masses, and tenderness.

c. High-pitched, harsh sound heard on inspiration when the trachea or larynx is obstructed.

d. Bluish or dark purple discoloration of the lips, skin, or nail beds.

e. Indirect measurement of cardiac output obtained by counting the number of peripheral pulse waves over a pulse point.

f. Low-pitched grating sound on inhalation and exhalation.

g. Respiratory rate greater than 24 beats per minute.

h. Abnormal, low-pitched breath sound, louder on exhalation.

i. Abnormal breath sound.

j. Abnormal breath sound that resembles a popping sound, heard in inhalation and exhalation, not cleared by coughing.

k. Review of the client's functional health patterns prior to the current contact with a health care agency.

l. Physical examination technique that involves listening to sounds in the body that are created by movement of air or fluid.

m. Heart rate less than 60 beats per minute in an adult.

n. Physical examination technique that uses short, tapping strokes on the surface of the skin to create vibrations of underlying organs.

___15. Hypoventilation

o. Condition in which the apical pulse rate is greater than the radial pulse rate.

___16. Inspection

p. Regularity of the heartbeat.

___17. Orthostatic Hypotension

q. Chart containing various-sized letters with standardized numbers at the end of each line of letters.

___18. Palpation

r. Brief account of any recent signs or symptoms related to any body system.

___19. Percussion

s. Medium-pitched and blowing sounds heard equally on inspiration and expiration from air moving through the large airways.

___20. Pleural Friction Rub

t. Easy respirations with a rate of breaths per minute that is age-appropriate.

___21. Pulse Amplitude

u. Outward expression of mood or emotions.

___22. Pulse Deficit

v. Respiratory rate of 10 or fewer breaths per minute.

___23. Pulse Rate

w. Physical examination technique that involves thorough visual observation.

___24. Pulse Rhythm

x. Heart rate in excess of 100 beats per minute in an adult.

___25. Review of Systems

y. Abnormal breath sound, high pitched and whistlelike in nature, during inhalation and exhalation.

___26. Sibilant Wheeze

z. Breathing characterized by shallow respirations.

___27. Snellen Chart

aa. Soft, breezy, low-pitched sound heard longer on inspiration than expiration that results from air moving through the smaller airways over the lung periphery, with the exception of the scapular area.

___28. Sonorous Wheeze

bb. Measurement of the strength or force exerted by the ejected blood against the arterial wall with each contraction.

___29. Stridor

cc. Difficulty breathing as observed by labored or forced respirations through the use of accessory muscles in the chest and neck.

___30. Tachycardia

dd. Loud, tubular, hollow-sounding breath sound normally heard over the sternum.

___31. Tachypnea

ee. Significant decrease in blood pressure that results in dizziness or lightheadedness when a person moves from a lying or sitting (supine) position to a standing position.

___32. Vesicular Sound

ff. Breathing characterized by deep, rapid respirations.

Abbreviation Review

Write the definition of the following abbreviations and acronyms.

1. AP _____
2. BP _____
3. cm _____
4. LLQ _____
5. LOC _____
6. LUQ _____
7. P _____
8. PERRLA _____
9. R _____
10. RLQ _____
11. ROS _____
12. RUQ _____
13. T _____

Exercises and Activities

1. What are the purposes of the health history and physical assessment?

   _____
   _____
   _____

   a. How can you establish rapport with your client?

      _____
      _____
      _____

   b. How can you provide comfort and privacy during the physical assessment?

      _____
      _____
      _____

   c. What findings might indicate that a client has been abused?

      _____
      _____
      _____

2. In which section of the health history would each of the following items be found?
   a. Completed hepatitis immunization _____
   b. Smokes one pack of cigarettes a day _____
   c. Last Pap test 6 months ago _____
   d. Experiencing stress from a new job _____

e. Client rates his health as an 8 on a scale of 1 to 10 _____

f. Sister and maternal grandmother have high blood pressure _____

g. Develops a rash with penicillin _____

h. "Began having severe stomach pain 1 hour ago" _____

i. Sleeps 7 hours a night, feels rested _____

j. Thyroidectomy at age 24 _____

k. Takes acetaminophen 650 mg q4h prn for headache _____

l. Chickenpox at age 5, no sequelae _____

3. Write at least two interventions that might be helpful for assessing each of the following clients.

An elderly client: _____

_____

A hearing-impaired client: _____

_____

A client who doesn't speak English: _____

_____

A client who is in pain: _____

_____

4. What items are included in the assessment of vital signs? Give normal findings for each.

_____

_____

_____

a. Why are vital signs an important part of an assessment?

_____

_____

_____

b. What factors can affect an individual's temperature?

_____

_____

_____

c. Convert the following temperatures:

97.7°F = _____ °C   38°C = _____ °F

101°F = _____ °C   39°C = _____ °F

d. Label and draw a line to each of the pulse points on the figure.

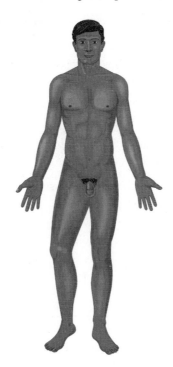

e. Draw an *X* over each area on this diagram where you would auscultate the lungs. Draw an arrow to show where you would assess the apical pulse.

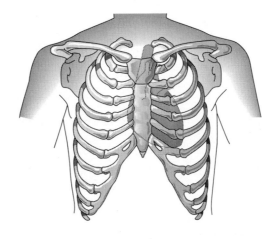

   f. Write a brief description of normal findings for an abdominal assessment on a client.

   _____

   _____

5. Mr. Moreno is a 71-year-old client with a history of cigarette smoking, obesity, hypertension, and diabetes mellitus. Vital signs are temperature 97.9°F, pulse 88, respirations 20, blood pressure 158/92, and a weight today of 213 lb. He is now exhibiting signs and symptoms of peripheral vascular disease, a complication of poorly controlled diabetes. During your assessment of the lower extremities, you note decreased leg hair, skin that is cool to touch, with some loss of sensation.

   a. What information from his health history might be helpful in planning nursing interventions and teaching for Mr. Moreno?

   _____

   _____

   _____

   _____

   b. Write three questions you could ask Mr. Moreno for the review of systems (ROS) for his legs.
      (1) _____
      (2) _____
      (3) _____

   c. What other information could you obtain during your physical examination of the legs?

   _____

   _____

   d. Where will you palpate the peripheral pulses for Mr. Moreno?

   _____

   _____

   e. Write two actual and two risk nursing diagnoses for this client.
      (1) _____
      (2) _____
      (3) _____
      (4) _____

   f. What elements will you include to complete the cardiovascular assessment on this client?

   _____

   _____

   _____

   _____

Self-Assessment Questions

Circle the letter that corresponds to the best answer for each question.

1. The nurse is performing percussion on the client's abdomen. If the assessment findings are normal, the nurse would note
   a. stridor.
   b. tympany.
   c. resonance.
   d. hyperresonance.

2. The nurse is preparing to do a physical assessment on an elderly client with difficulty breathing. Which position will the nurse use for respiratory assessment?
   a. Sims
   b. Supine
   c. Sitting
   d. Dorsal recumbent

3. An abdominal assessment finding that the nurse will report to a supervisor is
   a. positive borborygmi.
   b. audible peristalsis on auscultation.
   c. separation of the rectus abdominis muscle.
   d. finding abdominal organs with light palpation.

4. A nurse is performing a head and neck assessment on the client. To assess for visual acuity, the nurse will use
   a. a Snellen chart.
   b. direct light reflex.
   c. tangential lighting.
   d. an ophthalmoscope.

5. To accurately assess the apical pulse on the client, the nurse will
   a. palpate the brachial artery and count for 30 seconds.
   b. locate the left carotid artery and palpate gently for 1 minute.
   c. locate the fifth ICS, midclavicular line, and listen for 60 seconds.
   d. place the stethoscope on the left of the sternum and listen for 30 seconds.

6. The nurse is auscultating the lungs of a client with a respiratory illness. The breath sounds over the periphery of the lungs are normally described as
   a. resonant.
   b. vesicular.
   c. bronchial.
   d. hyperresonant.

Diagnostic Tests

Key Terms

Match the following terms with their correct definitions.

___ 1. Agglutination

___ 2. Agglutinin

___ 3. Agglutinogen

___ 4. Analyte

___ 5. Aneurysm

___ 6. Angiography

___ 7. Anion

___ 8. Antibody

___ 9. Antigen

___10. Arteriography

___11. Ascites

___12. Aspiration

___13. Bacteremia

___14. Barium

___15. Biopsy

___16. Cation

a. Visualization of the vascular structures through the use of fluoroscopy with a contrast medium.

b. Globular protein that is produced in the body and catalyzes chemical reactions within the cells by promoting the oxidative reactions and synthesis of various chemicals.

c. Blood in the urine.

d. Chalky-white contrast medium.

e. Venous catheter inserted into the superior vena cava through the subclavian or internal or external jugular vein.

f. Use of high-frequency sound waves to visualize deep body structures; also called an echogram.

g. Study of x-rays or gamma ray-exposed film through the action of ionizing radiation.

h. Diminished production of urine.

i. Minimally depressed level of consciousness during which the client retains the ability to maintain a continuously patent airway and to respond appropriately to physical stimulation or verbal commands.

j. Graphic recording of the heart's electrical activity.

k. Any antigenic substance that causes agglutination by the production of agglutinin.

l. Clumping together of red blood cells.

m. Immunoglobulin produced by the body in response to bacteria, viruses, or other antigenic substances.

n. Substance, usually a protein, that causes the formation of an antibody and reacts specifically with that antibody.

o. Excision of a small amount of tissue.

p. Product of incomplete fat metabolism.

___17. Central Line

q. Aspiration of cerebrospinal fluid from the subarachnoid space.

___18. Computed Tomography

r. Process of urine elimination.

___19. Conscious Sedation

s. Instrument that converts electrical energy to sound waves.

___20. Contrast Medium

t. Susceptibility of a pathogen to an antibiotic.

___21. Culture

u. Smear method of examining stained exfoliative cells.

___22. Cytology

v. Individual who performs venipuncture.

___23. Electrocardiogram

w. Radiopaque substance that facilitates roentgen (x-ray) imaging of the body's internal structures.

___24. Electroencephalogram

x. Specific kind of antibody whose interaction with antigens manifests as agglutination.

___25. Electrolyte

y. Procedure performed to withdraw fluid that has abnormally collected or to obtain a specimen.

___26. Endoscopy

z. Tissue death as the result of disease or injury.

___27. Enzyme

aa. Accessing body tissues, organs, or cavities through some type of instrumentation procedure.

___28. Fluoroscopy

bb. Colorless derivative of bilirubin formed by the normal bacterial action of intestinal flora on bilirubin.

___29. Hematuria

cc. Alert and with vital signs within the client's normal range.

___30. Invasive

dd. Aspiration of fluid from the abdominal cavity.

___31. Ketone

ee. Blood in the stool that can be detected only via a microscope or chemical means.

___32. Lipoprotein

ff. Radiological scanning of the body with x-ray beams and radiation detectors that transmit data to a computer that in turn transcribes the data into quantitative measurement and multidimensional images of the internal structures.

___33. Lumbar Puncture

gg. Descriptor for procedure wherein the body is not entered with any type of instrument.

___34. Magnetic Resonance Imaging

hh. Port that has been implanted under the skin with a catheter inserted into the superior vena cava or right atrium through the subclavian or internal jugular vein.

___35. Necrosis

ii. Immediate, serial images of the body's structure or function.

___36. Noninvasive

jj. Abnormal accumulation of fluid in the abdomen.

___37. Occult Blood

kk. Ion with a positive charge.

___38. Oliguria

ll. Weakness in the wall of a blood vessel.

___39. Papanicolaou Test

mm. Growing of microorganisms to identify a pathogen.

___40. Paracentesis

nn. Graphic recording of the brain's electrical activity.

___41. Phlebotomist

___42. Pneumothorax

___43. Port-a-Cath

___44. Radiography

___45. Sensitivity

___46. Stable

___47. Stress Test

___48. Thoracentesis

___49. Transducer

___50. Trocar

___51. Type and Cross-Match

___52. Ultrasound

___53. Urobilinogen

___54. Venipuncture

___55. Void

oo. Sharply pointed surgical instrument contained in a cannula.

pp. Visualization of a body organ or cavity through a scope.

qq. Puncturing of a vein with a needle to aspirate blood.

rr. Study of cells.

ss. Blood lipid bound to protein.

tt. Condition of bacteria in the blood.

uu. Ion with a negative charge.

vv. Substance that is measured.

ww. Substance that, when in solution, separates into ions and conducts electricity.

xx. Radiographic study of the vascular system following the injection of a radiopaque dye through a catheter.

yy. Condition wherein air or gas accumulates in the pleural space, causing the lungs to collapse.

zz. Measure of a client's cardiovascular response to exercise tolerance.

aaa. Laboratory test that identifies the client's blood type (e.g., A or B) and determines the compatibility of the blood between potential donor and recipient.

bbb. Aspiration of fluids from the pleural cavity.

ccc. Imaging technique that uses radio waves and a strong magnetic field to make continuous cross-sectional images of the body.

Abbreviation Review

Write the definition of the following abbreviations and acronyms.

1. ABG _____

2. C&S _____

3. CSF _____

4. CT _____

5. ECG (EKG) _____

6. EEG _____

7. HIV _____

8. I&O _____

9. IV _____

10. IVP _____

11. $PaCO_2$ _____

12. PaO_2 _____

13. RBC _____

14. WBC _____

Exercises and Activities

1. Describe the role of the nurse in preparing a client for diagnostic procedures.

_____

_____

_____

   a. What teaching will the nurse do with the client?

   _____

   _____

2. What is the role of the nurse during an invasive diagnostic procedure?

_____

_____

_____

   a. Why is it important to help the client relax or be comfortable during the procedure?

   _____

   _____

   b. How can the nurse help the client to be more relaxed?

   _____

   _____

   c. List ways to maintain safety for the nurse and the client during the procedure.

   _____

   _____

3. List normal values and identify the purpose of each of these common blood tests.

Test	*Normal Values*	*Purpose*
White blood cells (WBC)		
Hemoglobin (Hgb) and hematocrit (Hct)		
Arterial blood gas (ABG) analysis		
Serum electrolytes, Na^+ and K^+		
Fasting blood sugar (FBS)		

Test	*Normal Values*	*Purpose*
Glucose tolerance test (GTT)		
Blood urea nitrogen (BUN)		
Cholesterol (lipid profile)		

4. What documentation is the nurse responsible for following diagnostic procedures?

_____

_____

_____

5. For each of the following diagnostic procedures, briefly describe the purpose of the test, any special preparation for the client, and nursing assistance or interventions during the procedure.

Test	*Purpose*	*Preparation*	*Assistance*
Paracentesis			
Pap smear			
Cardiac catheterization			
Thoracentesis			
MRI			

6. Allen, a 19-year-old college sophomore, came to the hospital following the sudden onset of a severe headache, nausea and vomiting. On assessment he appears somewhat irritable, and displays stiffness in his neck. His temperature and pulse rate are increased, and he is breathing rapidly. One of the diagnostic tests that the physician has ordered is a lumbar puncture to rule out meningitis. Allen is extremely anxious and wants his friend to stay with him during the procedure.

a. How will you explain this procedure to Allen?

_____

_____

_____

b. What preparation is necessary?

_____

_____

_____

c. How will you assist the physician during the procedure?

_____

_____

_____

d. What are the normal laboratory values for this test?

_____

_____

_____

e. What can you do before and during the procedure to reduce Allen's anxiety?

_____

_____

_____

Self-Assessment Questions

Circle the letter that corresponds to the best answer for each question.

1. A nurse is caring for a client who is having an intravenous pyelogram (IVP). To monitor the client, the nurse should be aware that the most serious hazard of an allergic reaction to the dye is
   a. oliguria.
   b. urticaria.
   c. respiratory distress.
   d. low blood pressure.

2. A practitioner has ordered a urine sample for a creatinine clearance test. The most appropriate method to collect this is from a
   a. timed sample.
   b. sterile specimen.
   c. random collection.
   d. clean-voided specimen.

3. A nurse is caring for a client who has experienced a bronchoscopy. Following this procedure, it is important for the nurse to
   a. observe the client for signs of tachycardia.
   b. withhold fluids until the gag reflex returns.
   c. advise the client that he may experience dysphagia.
   d. place the client in a high Fowler's position to minimize coughing.

4. The nurse is aware that the most serious complication of thoracentesis is
    a. dyspnea.
    b. infection.
    c. dysrhythmia.
    d. pneumothorax.

5. A client is recovering after having a cardiac catheterization. Following this procedure, it is important for the client to
    a. maintain a side-lying position with the knees bent.
    b. limit fluid intake for several hours until the medication has worn off.
    c. keep the extremity in which the catheter was placed straight and immobile.
    d. collect urine for 24 hours for proper disposal related to the use of radiographic dyes.

6. The nurse correctly describes conscious sedation to the client as
    a. a state of relaxation using biofeedback techniques.
    b. anesthesia delivered by a nurse working in an "expanded role."
    c. a state where the client is awake and aware but unable to move.
    d. a depressed level of consciousness in which the client can breathe on his own.

Pain Management

Key Terms

Match the following terms with their correct definitions.

___ 1. Acupuncture

   a. Discomfort identified by sudden onset and relatively short duration, mild to severe intensity, and a steady decrease in intensity over several days or weeks.

___ 2. Acute Pain

   b. Discomfort that occurs almost daily, has been present for at least 6 months, and ranges in intensity from mild to severe; also known as chronic benign pain.

___ 3. Adjuvant Medication

   c. Descending spinal cord pathway that transmits sensory impulses from the brain.

___ 4. Afferent Pain Pathway

   d. Neuropathic pain that occurs after amputation with pain sensations referred to an area in the missing portion of the limb.

___ 5. Analgesia

   e. Unpleasant sensory and emotional experience associated with actual or potential tissue damage or described in terms of such.

___ 6. Analgesic

   f. Compound that blocks opioid effects on one receptor type while producing opioid effects on a second receptor type.

___ 7. Ceiling Effect

   g. Drug used to enhance the analgesic efficacy of opioids, treat concurrent symptoms that exacerbate pain, and provide independent analgesia for specific types of pain.

___ 8. Chronic Acute Pain

   h. Use of cold applications to reduce swelling.

___ 9. Chronic Nonmalignant Pain

   i. Analgesics administered via a catheter that terminates in the epidural space.

___10. Chronic Pain

   j. Technique of focusing attention on stimuli other than pain.

___11. Colic

   k. State of heightened awareness and focused concentration.

___12. Cryotherapy

   l. Discomfort from the internal organs that is felt in another area of the body.

___13. Cutaneous Pain

___14. Distraction

___15. Efferent Pain Pathway

___16. Endorphins

___17. Epidural Analgesia

___18. Gate Control Pain Theory

___19. Hypnosis

___20. Intrathecal Analgesia

___21. Ischemic Pain

___22. Mixed Agonist-Antagonist

___23. Modulation

___24. Myofascial Pain Syndromes

___25. Neuralgia

___26. Nociceptor

___27. Noxious Stimulus

___28. Pain

___29. Pain Threshold

___30. Pain Tolerance

___31. Patient-Controlled Analgesia

m. Stress management strategy in which muscles are alternately tensed and relaxed.

n. Underlying pathology that causes pain.

o. Central nervous system pathway that selectively inhibits pain transmission by sending signals back down to the dorsal horn of the spinal cord.

p. Paroxysmal pain that extends along the course of one or more nerves.

q. Noxious stimulus that triggers electrical activity in the endings of afferent nerve fibers (nociceptors).

r. Process of applying a low-voltage electrical current to the skin through cutaneous electrodes.

s. Phenomenon of requiring larger and larger doses of an analgesic to achieve the same level of pain relief.

t. Discomfort resulting when the blood supply of an area is restricted or cut off completely.

u. Level of intensity at which a person feels pain.

v. Usually delivered by a device that allows the client to control the delivery of intravenous or subcutaneous pain medication in a safe, effective manner through a programmable pump.

w. Discomfort marked by repetitive painful episodes that may recur over a prolonged period or throughout a client's lifetime.

x. Technique of monitoring negative thoughts and replacing them with positive ones.

y. Discomfort caused by stimulation of the cutaneous nerve endings in the skin.

z. Group of opiate-like substances produced naturally by the brain; these substances raise the pain threshold, produce sedation and euphoria, and promote a sense of well-being.

aa. Pain relief without producing anesthesia.

bb. Ascending spinal cord that transmits sensory impulses to the brain.

cc. Administration of analgesics into the subarachnoid space.

dd. Receptive neuron for painful sensations.

ee. Nonlocalized discomfort originating in tendons, ligaments, and nerves.

___32. Perception

ll. Theory that proposes that the cognitive, sensory, emotional, and physiological components of the body can act together to block an individual's perception of pain.

___33. Phantom Limb Pain

ff. Level of intensity or duration of pain that a person is willing to endure.

___34. Progressive Muscle Relaxation

gg. Discomfort generally identified as long term (lasting 6 months or longer) that is persistent, nearly constant, or recurrent and that produces significant negative changes in a person's life.

___35. Recurrent Acute Pain

hh. Insertion of small needles into the skin at selected (hoku) sites.

___36. Referred Pain

ii. Substance that relieves pain.

___37. Reframing

jj. Condition of acute abdominal pain.

___38. Relaxation Technique

kk. Discomfort that occurs almost daily over a long period, has the potential for lasting months or years, and has a high probability of ending; also known as progressive pain.

___39. Somatic Pain

mm. Group of muscle disorders characterized by pain, muscle spasm, tenderness, stiffness, and limited motion.

___40. Tolerance

nn. Process whereby the pain impulse travels from the receiving nociceptors to the spinal cord.

___41. Transcutaneous Electrical Nerve Stimulation

oo. Method used to decrease anxiety and muscle tension.

___42. Transduction

pp. Discomfort felt in the internal organs.

___43. Transmission

qq. Ability to experience, recognize, organize, and interpret sensory stimuli.

___44. Visceral Pain

rr. Medication dosage beyond which no further analgesia occurs.

Abbreviation Review

Write the definition of the following abbreviations and acronyms.

1. APS _____

2. AHCPR _____

3. ATC _____

4. EMLA _____

5. HCl _____

6. IASP _____

7. mcg _____

8. MRI _____

9. NPO _____

10. NSAID _____

11. PCA _____

12. po _____

13. prn _____

14. q _____

15. SC/SQ _____

16. TAC _____

17. TENS _____

18. TMJ _____

19. VAS _____

20. WHO _____

Exercises and Activities

1. In what ways is the role of the nurse important in pain relief?

   _____

   _____

   _____

   _____

   _____

   _____

   a. What is the importance of pain control to an individual's health?

   _____

   _____

   _____

   _____

   b. Why has chronic pain been called "a disease state"?

   _____

   _____

   _____

   _____

   c. How can pain be a diagnostic tool?

   _____

   _____

   _____

   _____

2. Draw and label the pain pathway from the stimulus to the muscle response.

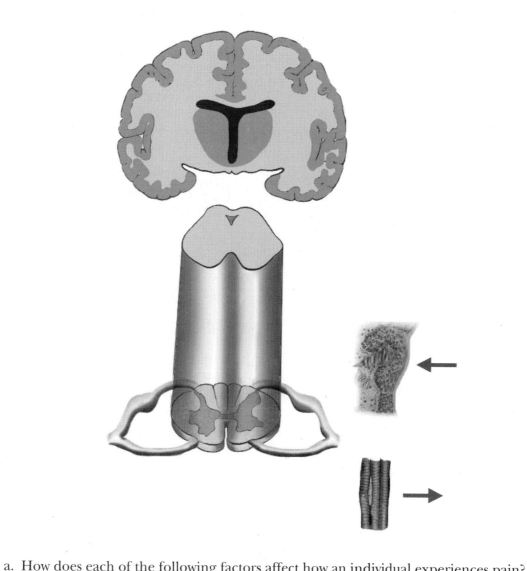

a. How does each of the following factors affect how an individual experiences pain?

Their age: _____

_____

Previous experiences with pain: _____

_____

Cultural norms: _____

_____

The meaning/implications of the pain: _____

_____

b. Briefly describe the three general principles of pain management.

(1)_____

(2)_____

(3)_____

3. How can you determine the amount of pain your client is experiencing?

_____

_____

_____

a. Compare and give examples for the three categories of pain control interventions.

Category	Examples	Advantages	Disadvantages
Pharmacological			
Noninvasive			
Invasive			

b. How do nonopioid analgesics differ from opioid analgesics?

_____

_____

c. What are the nurse's responsibilities in administration of analgesics?

_____

_____

4. A client gives the following description of a headache:

"About 2 hours ago I started getting this awful headache right in the back of my head, just above my neck. I've had plenty of headaches before, but this one just came on with no warning, and now it feels like someone is pounding a hammer inside my head. I started feeling sick to my stomach and even vomited a couple of times. All I had at home to take for the headache was some mild pain medicine, but it didn't even touch the pain. Since my mother died a couple of years ago from a stroke, every headache I get really worries me."

a. What subjective and objective information would be helpful to assess this client's level of pain?

_____

_____

b. For a complete description of the pain, list at least five specific questions will you ask this client.

(1) _____

(2) _____

(3) _____

(4) _____

(5) _____

c. What terms might clients use to describe the "quality" of their pain?

_____

_____

5. Mrs. Lindstrom is a 34-year-old client who had an amputation of her right leg below the knee as a result of extensive trauma 3 years ago. Since then, she has experienced chronic neuropathic pain ranging from mild to moderate. With a prosthesis, she is able to care for her family and do housework, but she has difficulty sitting for extended periods of time or walking long distances. Mrs. Lindstrom has tried several types of pain medication over the past year but states that the ones that give enough relief make her feel too sleepy.

a. What type of pain is Mrs. Lindstrom experiencing?

_____

_____

b. List five ways in which the pain Mrs. Lindstrom is experiencing differs from acute pain.

(1) _____

(2) _____

(3) _____

(4) _____

(5) _____

c. Does this client's pain serve as a protective mechanism?

_____

_____

d. Mrs. Lindstrom says that she would like to try something to help ease her pain besides just medication. Suggest two interventions and explain your rationale.

(1) _____

_____

_____

(2) _____

_____

_____

e. Why will she need ongoing pain assessments?

_____

_____

_____

_____

Self-Assessment Questions

Circle the letter that corresponds to the best answer for each question.

1. To reverse respiratory depression in a client receiving Duramorph, the nurse would administer
   a. naloxone.
   b. an amphetamine.
   c. an opioid agonist.
   d. a neurolytic agent.

2. The nurse is assessing a client's level of pain 2 days postsurgery. The most effective way for the nurse to determine the client's pain level is to
   a. evaluate the amount of pain medication taken.
   b. ask the client to describe her perception of the pain.
   c. assess the client's mobility and level of self-care activities.
   d. note the facial expressions and the presence of guarding.

3. As part of a comprehensive pain management plan, noninvasive interventions may include relaxation techniques, guided imagery, distraction, and
   a. radiation.
   b. cryotherapy.
   c. nerve blocks.
   d. nonopioid analgesia.

4. The primary advantage of using patient-controlled analgesia (PCA) is that it
   a. has fewer systemic side effects.
   b. can be used in the home setting.
   c. gives clients greater control over their pain.
   d. uses lower doses of medication to achieve pain relief.

5. A nurse is caring for a client who continues to experience neck and back pain following an automobile accident 1 year ago. Because of the chronic pain, this client is most likely to
   a. use analgesic medication effectively.
   b. display signs that resemble those of anxiety.
   c. exhibit the same behaviors as a client in acute pain.
   d. benefit from nonpharmacological pain relief methods..

Anesthesia

Key Terms

Match the following terms with their correct definitions.

___ 1. Amnesia

___ 2. Analgesia

___ 3. Anesthesia

___ 4. Anesthesiologist

___ 5. Anesthetist

___ 6. General Anesthesia

___ 7. Orthostatic Hypotension

___ 8. Regional Anesthesia

___ 9. Sedation

___10. Synergism

a. Method of producing unconsciousness; complete insensibility to pain; amnesia; motionlessness; and muscle relaxation.

b. Inability to remember things.

c. Method of temporarily rendering a region of the body insensible to pain.

d. Significant decrease in blood pressure that results when a person moves from a lying or sitting (supine) position to a standing position.

e. Result of two or more agents working together to achieve a greater effect than either could produce alone.

f. Qualified RN, dentist, or medical doctor who administers anesthetics.

g. Pain relief without producing anesthesia.

h. Licensed physician educated and skilled in the delivery of anesthesia who also adds to the knowledge of anesthesia through research or other scholarly pursuits.

i. Absence of the sensation of pain.

j. Reduction of stress, excitement, or irritability via some degree of central nervous system depression.

Abbreviation Review

Write the definition of the following abbreviations and acronyms.

1. cc _____

2. CNS _____

3. CRNA _____

4. CSF _____

5. ETT _____

6. HR _____

7. NSAID _____

8. PCA _____

9. PDPH _____

Exercises and Activities

1. Describe the role of the nurse in providing care to a client before surgery.

   _____

   _____

   _____

   a. Medications that may be administered prior to surgery include:

      _____

      _____

   b. List at least five items that must be documented in the client's chart before surgery.

      (1) _____

      (2) _____

      (3) _____

      (4) _____

      (5) _____

   c. Why are oral fluids and food normally withheld before surgery?

      _____

      _____

2. What is the difference between sedation and general anesthesia?

   _____

   _____

   _____

   a. What client monitoring is needed during sedation?

      _____

      _____

   b. In what ways might a client's anxiety and pain affect the medication required before and during surgery?

      _____

      _____

   c. Describe the recovery phase from general anesthesia related to the following factors:

      Oxygenation/ventilation:

      _____

      _____

Heart rate and blood pressure:

_____

_____

  d. List five factors that can contribute to a client's hypothermia or shivering.

    (1) _____

    (2) _____

    (3) _____

    (4) _____

    (5) _____

  e. List three factors that could contribute to fluid imbalance during surgery.

    (1) _____

    (2) _____

    (3) _____

3. Briefly describe the following methods of postoperative pain management and give at least one advantage and disadvantage or risk for each.

Pain Management	Description	Advantages	Disadvantages/Risks
PCA			
Regional analgesia			
Opioids			

4. Mr. Reid is a 31-year-old client who is having a surgical repair to his left knee. Three months ago, while on a skiing trip, Mr. Reid suffered an acute injury to his left anterior cruciate ligament (ACL) that provides support for the knee. Since the accident, he has experienced pain and loss of function in the joint. His physician has determined that ACL reconstruction will be beneficial. Although he is apprehensive, Mr. Reid is glad that having epidural anesthesia will allow him to be awake during the surgery.

  a. While Mr. Reid is being prepared for surgery, his wife asks you what an "epidural" is. How could you explain it to her?

_____

_____

_____

b. What preparation will be needed before an epidural is administered?

_____

_____

_____

c. Mr. Reid has had asthma for many years. How might an epidural block be safer than general anesthesia for him?

_____

_____

_____

d. What types of residual effects might be noted as the anesthetic wears off following his surgery?

_____

_____

_____

e. What symptoms would indicate that Mr. Reid might be experiencing a postdural puncture headache (PDPH)? What would treatment include?

_____

_____

_____

Self-Assessment Questions

Circle the letter that corresponds to the best answer for each question.

1. Following general anesthesia, the ability of the client to respond to verbal commands and maintain his own airway are indicators of
   a. complete recovery.
   b. residual sensory block.
   c. skeletal muscle contraction.
   d. the initial phase of emergence.

2. The anesthetic most commonly used for epidural blocks is
   a. Epicaine.
   b. Marcaine.
   c. Xylocaine.
   d. Sublimaze.

3. A client has received regional anesthesia for a surgical procedure. Because the sympathetic nerves are the last type of nerve to recover, the client may experience
   a. an abnormal heart rate.
   b. orthostatic hypotension.
   c. increased pain sensation.
   d. blood pressure elevation.

4. Which of the following drugs may be used for surgical procedures that require the client to have complete skeletal muscle relaxation?
   a. Pavulon
   b. Xylocaine
   c. Prostigmin
   d. Carbocaine

5. The nurse is caring for a client who is experiencing a postdural puncture headache. Interventions will include all except which of the following?
   a. Analgesics
   b. Increased IV fluids
   c. Epidural blood patch
   d. Ambulation with assistance

6. The client is recovering from an epidural block anesthesia that included a long-acting opioid. During assessment, the nurse notes that the client has a respiratory rate of 10 breaths/minute. The best action for the nurse is to
   a. initiate CPR.
   b. notify the anesthesia provider.
   c. record normal emergence from anesthesia.
   d. continue monitoring respiratory rate and blood pressure.

Nursing Care of the Surgical Client

Key Terms

Match the following terms with their correct definitions.

___ 1. Aldrete Score

    a. Associate of the surgeon, referring physician, or surgical resident who assists the surgeon to retract tissue, aids in the removal of blood and fluids at the operative site, and assists with hemostasis and wound closure.

___ 2. Ambulatory Surgery

    b. Time during the surgical experience that begins when the client is transferred to the operating room table and ends when the client is admitted to the postanesthesia care unit.

___ 3. Asepsis

    c. Time during the surgical experience that begins at the end of the surgical procedure and ends when the client is discharged from medical care by the surgeon in addition to being discharged from the hospital or institution.

___ 4. Aseptic Technique

    d. RN responsible and accountable for management of personnel, equipment, supplies, the environment, and communication throughout a surgical procedure.

___ 5. Circulating Nurse

    e. Area surrounding the client and the surgical site that is free from all microorganisms; created by draping of the work area and the client with sterile drapes.

___ 6. Dehiscence

    f. RN, LP/VN, or surgical technologist who provides services under the direction of the circulating nurse and who is qualified by training or experience to prepare and maintain the integrity, safety, and efficiency of the sterile field throughout an operation.

___ 7. Evisceration

    g. Surgical operation performed under general, regional, or local anesthesia and involving fewer than 24 hours of hospitalization.

___ 8. First Assistant

    h. Treatment of injury, disease, or deformity through invasive operative methods.

___ 9. Informed Consent

    i. Complication of wound healing wherein the wound edges and layers separate below the skin.

___10. Intraoperative Phase

j. Legal form signed by a competent client and witnessed by another person that grants permission to the client's physician to perform the procedure described by the physician and that demonstrates the client's understanding of the benefits, risks, and possible complications of the procedure, as well as alternate treatment options.

___11. Perioperative

k. Without microorganisms.

___12. Postoperative Phase

l. Scoring system for objectively assessing the physical status of clients recovering from anesthesia; serves as a basis for dismissal from the postanesthesia care unit (PACU) and ambulatory surgery; also known as the postanesthetic recovery score.

___13. Preoperative Phase

m. Period of time comprising the preoperative, intraoperative, and postoperative phases of surgery.

___14. Scrub Nurse

n. Complication of wound healing characterized by a complete separation of wound edges accompanied by visceral protrusion.

___15. Sterile

o. Collection of principles used to control and/or prevent the transfer of pathogenic microorganisms from sources within (endogenous) and outside (exogenous) the client.

___16. Sterile Conscience

p. Time during the surgical experience that begins when the client decides to have surgery and ends when the client is transferred to the operating table.

___17. Sterile Field

q. Individual's personal sense of honesty and integrity with regard to adherence to the principles of aseptic technique, including prompt admission and correction of any errors and omissions.

___18. Surgery

r. Absence of pathogenic microorganisms.

Abbreviation Review

Write the definition of the following abbreviations and acronyms.

1. ALT _____
2. AORN _____
3. AST _____
4. BUN _____
5. CRNA _____
6. DO _____
7. EENT _____
8. ESU _____
9. ET _____
10. Hct _____

11. Hgb _____

12. L _____

13. MAO _____

14. mL _____

15. MD _____

16. OR _____

17. PACU _____

18. PT _____

19. PTT _____

20. RNFA _____

Exercises and Activities

1. Why is a thorough preoperative nursing assessment essential for the surgical client?

   _____

   _____

   _____

   a. Identify the sources of data for a nursing preoperative assessment.

      _____

      _____

   b. Why is the evaluation of the client's psychological well-being important?

      _____

      _____

   c. List three of the most common fears of clients who are facing surgery.

      (1) _____

      (2) _____

      (3) _____

   d. What signs and symptoms can indicate anxiety in the client?

      _____

      _____

   e. List the four purposes of preoperative teaching.

      (1) _____

      (2) _____

      (3) _____

      (4) _____

2. What items and preparation need to be documented before a surgical procedure?

   _____

   _____

   _____

a. Why are renal and hepatic status in the client important?

_____

_____

b. What factors in a client's medical history increase the risk for infection?

_____

_____

c. List specific preoperative activities that prepare the client the morning of surgery.

_____

_____

_____

3. Identify items and procedures that promote asepsis in the surgical suite.

_____

_____

_____

a. Describe the concept of a "sterile conscience."

_____

_____

b. How would you instruct another student to perform a surgical hand scrub?

_____

_____

_____

_____

c. Identify each of the following figures:

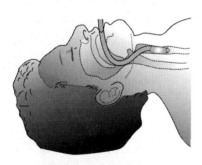

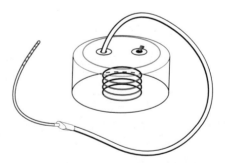

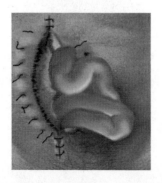

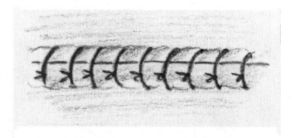

4. How will the nurse in the postanesthesia care unit (PACU) monitor a client's respiratory and cardiovascular status?

_____

_____

_____

a. List five signs of respiratory distress.

(1) _____

(2) _____

(3) _____

(4) _____

(5) _____

b. Why is the postoperative client at risk for aspiration?

_____

_____

c. What observations and care are required for the surgical wound dressing and any drains?

_____

_____

_____

_____

5. Mr. O'Quinn, a 70-year-old client, has been admitted from a long-term care facility where he has been a resident for the past 3 weeks. He is now scheduled for a lower extremity amputation related to long-term peripheral vascular disease, a result of his diabetes. At first, Mr. O'Quinn refused surgery, saying he was "just going to die anyway," but he recently decided to have the procedure done, after strong encouragement from his family. During the preoperative assessment, the nurse notes that Mr. O'Quinn is moderately anxious and shows signs of poor nutrition and skin breakdown from his lack of mobility. His wife mentions that he has a hearing aid with him but doesn't like to use it.

a. What items will the nurse include in Mr. O'Quinn's preoperative teaching? How might his anxiety affect his ability to learn?

_____

_____

_____

b. What complications do elderly clients have associated with surgical procedures?

_____

_____

_____

c. Because Mr. O'Quinn is diabetic and insulin-dependent, what complications is he at risk for developing?

_____

_____

_____

d. Identify four risk nursing diagnoses for this client.

(1) _____

(2) _____

(3) _____

(4) _____

e. Identify nursing interventions that will help prevent skin breakdown during and after surgery.

_____

_____

f. What factors are present for Mr. O'Quinn that could delay wound healing?

_____

_____

_____

_____

Self-Assessment Questions

Circle the letter that corresponds to the best answer for each question.

1. The nurse is caring for ambulatory (same-day) surgery clients. Which of the following actions by the nurse will be most important in preventing nosocomial infection?
    a. Using aseptic technique
    b. Administering antibiotics prophylactically
    c. Having the client cough and deep breathe
    d. Teaching the client about ways to prevent infection

2. The postoperative phase of recovery for the client begins when the surgical procedure is completed and lasts until the client is
    a. well enough to be discharged home.
    b. fully recovered from the effects of anesthesia.
    c. discharged from medical care by the surgeon.
    d. returned to the general medical-surgical unit from PACU.

3. To assess renal function in the preoperative client, the physician orders a
    a. urine C&S.
    b. PTT and APTT.
    c. 24-hour urine collection.
    d. BUN and serum creatinine.

4. The nurse is caring for a postoperative client who now has an Aldrete Score of 10. Based on this information, the nurse will
   a. administer pain medication.
   b. likely transfer the client from PACU.
   c. notify the physician about the client's respiratory depression.
   d. continue monitoring the client every 15 minutes until a score of 20 is achieved.

5. Because of the effects of medication, a neurological assessment for the postoperative client does not include the client's
   a. level of consciousness.
   b. ability to answer questions.
   c. responsiveness to verbal stimulation.
   d. orientation to person, place, and time.

6. A nurse is preparing to instruct the client on postoperative care to be done at home. The best time for the nurse to begin teaching is
   a. at the time of the client's admission.
   b. immediately after the surgical procedure.
   c. when family members arrive to take the client home.
   d. after the client has received medication for pain and nausea.

7. The nurse is caring for an elderly client 1 day after surgery. Because this client is at risk for atelectasis, the nurse will
   a. maintain the client on supplemental oxygen.
   b. limit fluid intake to decrease fluid in the lungs.
   c. limit pain medication to prevent respiratory depression.
   d. instruct the client to cough, deep breathe, and move often.

8. The nurse is performing an assessment on a client who is recovering from abdominal surgery. Which of these findings by the nurse may indicate an impending wound dehiscence?
   a. Abdominal distension
   b. Sudden increase in drainage
   c. The client's statement of pain
   d. Low-grade fever and tachycardia

Nursing Care of the Oncology Client

![image]

Key Terms

Match the following terms with their correct definitions.

___ 1. Alopecia

___ 2. Anorexia

___ 3. Antineoplastic

___ 4. Benign

___ 5. Biologic Response Modifier

___ 6. Cachexia

___ 7. Cancer

___ 8. Carcinogen

___ 9. Carcinoma

___10. Chemotherapy

___11. Curative

___12. Differentiation

___13. Extravasation

___14. Leukemia

___15. Lymphoma

___16. Malignant

___17. Metastasis

___18. Neoplasm

___19. Oncology

___20. Palliative

___21. Radiotherapy

a. State of malnutrition and protein wasting.

b. Cancer occurring in infection-fighting organs.

c. Agent that may produce blisters and tissue necrosis.

d. Loss of appetite.

e. To heal or restore to health.

f. Cancer occurring in blood-forming tissues.

g. Not progressive; favorable for recovery.

h. Partial or complete baldness or loss of hair.

i. Disease resulting from the uncontrolled growth of cells, which causes malignant cellular tumors.

j. Acquisition of functions different from those of the original kind.

k. Spread of cancer cells to distant areas of the body by way of the lymph system or bloodstream.

l. To rebuild or reestablish.

m. Any abnormal growth of new tissue.

n. Escape of fluid into the surrounding tissue.

o. Use of drugs to treat illness, especially cancer.

p. Agent that destroys malignant cells by stimulating the body's immune system.

q. Agent that inhibits the growth and reproduction of malignant cells.

r. Cancer occurring in epithelial tissue.

s. Becoming progressively worse and often resulting in death.

t. Relief of symptoms, such as pain, without altering the course of disease.

u. Substance found in the serum that indicates the possible presence of malignancy.

___22. Reconstructive

v. Study of tumors.

___23. Sarcoma

w. Substance that initiates or promotes the development of cancer.

___24. Stomatitis

x. Treatment of cancer with high-energy radiation.

___25. Tumor Marker

y. Cancer occurring in connective tissue.

___26. Vesicant

z. Inflammation of the mucous membrane of the oral cavity.

Abbreviation Review

Write the definition of the following abbreviations and acronyms.

1. ACS _____

2. AHCPR _____

3. BCG _____

4. BMT _____

5. CCNS _____

6. CCS _____

7. CNS _____

8. CT _____

9. DNA _____

10. EPA _____

11. EVAD _____

12. IVAD _____

13. OSHA _____

14. RNA _____

15. TENS _____

16. TNM _____

17. TPN _____

Exercises and Activities

1. How do cancer cells differ from normal cells?

_____

_____

_____

a. Describe how tumor markers help in cancer detection.

_____

_____

b. How does staging of tumors differ from grading of tumors?

_____

_____

c. What is a stage II tumor?

_____

_____

2. List the lifestyle factors that may increase an individual's risk for cancer.

_____

_____

_____

a. According to Table 17-1, smoking is a risk factor for which types of cancer?

_____

_____

b. You are asked to present a class to women on healthy behaviors. What would you include in your teaching to help them lower their risk for cancer? What recommendations would you make for health screening for early detection?

_____

_____

_____

_____

3. How are palliative and reconstructive surgery used in the treatment of cancer?

_____

_____

_____

a. Describe how each of these treatments destroys cancer cells.

Radiation: _____

_____

Chemotherapy: _____

_____

Biotherapy: _____

_____

Bone marrow transplantation: _____

_____

b. What precautions are important for health care workers when a client is treated with radiation?

_____

_____

c. Identify the cause and three nursing interventions for the following complications.

Problem	Cause	Interventions
Bone marrow dysfunction		(1) (2) (3)
Poor nutrition		(1) (2) (3)
Fatigue		(1) (2) (3)
Dyspnea		(1) (2) (3)
Ascites		(1) (2) (3)

d. List four medical emergencies that can develop with advanced cancer.

(1) _____

(2) _____

(3) _____

(4) _____

4. Mrs. Russell, a 72-year-old client, has been admitted to your unit following a collapse in her apartment. Although usually in good health, she had noticed increasing fatigue and leg pain with a lesion developing on the right lower leg. After feeling ill all morning, she attempted to stand up, but sudden, severe leg pain and general weakness caused her to fall, hitting her head. A neighbor found her the next day, and she was admitted to the hospital. Mrs. Russell has now been diagnosed with multiple myeloma, a malignancy affecting the bone marrow and soft tissue. She has refused surgery but is undergoing radiation. Mrs. Russell has very limited mobility and weight-bearing on her right side. During your morning care, you note two large, draining, purplish-red lesions on her right leg, two new discolored areas on her left leg, and one on her back. Pressure on her right leg causes a great deal of pain, and she now has very little appetite.

a. List four actual nursing diagnoses for this client.

(1) _____

(2) _____

(3) _____

(4) _____

b. Circle the nursing diagnosis in the preceding list that you believe is most important, and identify at least three nursing interventions.

(1) _____

(2) _____

(3) _____

c. What side effects of radiation do you need to monitor for?

_____

_____

d. What impact can pain have on the client with cancer?

_____

_____

_____

_____

e. Because Mrs. Russell is most likely in an advanced stage of cancer, what are your goals for her?

_____

_____

_____

_____

Self-Assessment Questions

Circle the letter that corresponds to the best answer for each question.

1. A nurse is caring for a client with breast cancer. Because the cancer has metastasized to the bone, the nurse will monitor for signs and symptoms of which serious complication?
   a. Hypokalemia
   b. Osteomyelitis
   c. Hypercalcemia
   d. Spinal cord compression

2. Your client is exposed to vinyl chloride, a carcinogen, at his job. Because of his occupational exposure, you will include in your health teaching that it is especially important for him to
   a. lose weight.
   b. stop smoking.
   c. avoid alcohol.
   d. take vitamin supplements.

3. For the client with cancer that has metastasized, palliative surgery may be used to
   a. restore health.
   b. relieve symptoms.
   c. minimize deformity.
   d. improve the survival rate.

4. You are caring for a client with pancreatic cancer. Because he is showing signs of cachexia, you determine that your client would most benefit from
   a. antibiotics.
   b. pain control.
   c. oxygen therapy.
   d. nutritional guidance.

5. A nursing student is assigned to care for a client with a grade IV tumor. Based on this information, the instructor explains to the student that this client's tumor
   a. involves at least four lymph nodes.
   b. is most responsive to chemotherapy.
   c. is undifferentiated with a poor prognosis.
   d. involves metastasis to another organ or bone.

Nursing Care of the Client: Respiratory System

Key Terms

Match the following terms with their correct definitions.

___ 1. Adventitious Breath Sound

___ 2. Asthma

___ 3. Atelectasis

___ 4. Audible Wheeze

___ 5. Bronchial Breath Sound

___ 6. Bronchiectasis

___ 7. Bronchitis

___ 8. Bronchovesicular Breath Sound

___ 9. Caseation

___ 10. Cavitation

___ 11. Chemoreceptor

___ 12. Coarse Crackle

___ 13. Diffusion

___ 14. Emphysema

___ 15. Epistaxis

___ 16. External Respiration

___ 17. Fine Crackle

a. Lung disease wherein air accumulates in the tissues of the lungs.

b. Condition wherein blood accumulates in the pleural space of the lungs.

c. Persistent, intractable asthma attack.

d. Condition wherein air or gas accumulates in the pleural space of the lungs, causing the lungs to collapse.

e. Condition characterized by intermittent airway obstruction due to antigen antibody reaction.

f. Receptor that monitors the levels of carbon dioxide, oxygen, and pH in the blood.

g. Abnormal sound, including sibilant wheezes (formerly wheezes), sonorous wheezes (formerly rhonchi), fine and coarse crackles (formerly rales), and pleural friction rubs.

h. Inflammation of the bronchioles and alveoli accompanied by consolidation, or solidification of exudate, in the lungs.

i. Collection of pleural fluid within the pleural cavity.

j. Process of exchanging oxygen and carbon dioxide.

k. Phospholipid that is present in the lungs and lowers surface tension to prevent collapse of the airways.

l. Breath sound normally heard in the area of the scapula and near the sternum; medium in pitch and intensity, with inspiratory and expiratory phases of equal length.

m. Lung disorder characterized by chronic dilation of the bronchi.

n. Exchange of gases between the atmosphere and the lungs.

o. Exchange of oxygen and carbon dioxide at the cellular level.

p. Movement of air into and out of the lungs.

q. Death and subsequent change of tissue to a liquid or semi-liquid state; often descriptive of a primary tubercle.

___18. Hemopneumothorax

r. Abnormal breath sound that is low pitched and snoring in nature and is louder on expiration.

___19. Hemothorax

s. Nodule that contains tubercle bacilli and forms within lung tissue.

___20. Internal Respiration

t. Condition arising from inflammation of the pleura, or sac, that encases the lung.

___21. Liquefaction Necrosis

u. Abnormal breath sound that is creaky and grating in nature and is heard on inspiration and expiration.

___22. Lung Stretch Receptor

v. Receptor that monitors the patterns of breathing and prevents overexpansion of the lungs.

___23. Perfusion

w. Collapse of a lung or a portion of a lung.

___24. Pleural Effusion

x. Wheeze that can be heard without the aid of a stethoscope.

___25. Pleural Friction Rub

y. Inflammation of the bronchial tree accompanied by hypersecretion of mucus.

___26. Pleurisy

z. Process whereby the center of the primary tubercle formed in the lungs as a result of tuberculosis becomes soft and cheeselike due to decreased perfusion.

___27. Pneumonia

aa. Process whereby a cavity is created in the lung tissue through the liquefaction and rupture of a primary tubercle.

___28. Pneumothorax

bb. Moist, low-pitched crackling and gurgling lung sound of long duration.

___29. Primary Tubercle

cc. Hemorrhage of the nares or nostrils; also known as nosebleed.

___30. Respiration

dd. Dry, high-pitched crackling and popping lung sound of short duration.

___31. Sibilant Wheeze

ee. Abnormal breath sound that is high pitched and musical in nature and is heard on inhalation and exhalation.

___32. Sonorous Wheeze

ff. Blood flow through an organ or body part.

___33. Status Asthmaticus

gg. Loud, tubular, hollow-sounding breath sound normally heard over the sternum.

___34. Stridor

hh. Process whereby a substance moves from an area of higher concentration to an area of lower concentration.

___35. Surfacant

ii. Soft, low breath sound heard over the majority of lung tissue.

___36. Ventilation

jj. Condition wherein blood and air accumulate in the pleural space of the lungs.

___37. Vesicular Breath Sound

kk. Abnormal breath sound that is crowing in nature and is louder on inspiration.

Abbreviation Review

Write the meaning or definition of the following abbreviations, acronyms, and symbols.

1. ABG _____

2. AFB _____

3. APTT _____

4. ARDS _____

5. ASO _____

6. BCG _____

7. CAL _____

8. CAT _____

9. CHF _____

10. CO_2 _____

11. COLD _____

12. COPD _____

13. CT _____

14. CVA _____

15. H^+ _____

16. H_2CO_3 _____

17. HCO_3^- _____

18. INH _____

19. INR _____

20. IV _____

21. L _____

22. mEq/L _____

23. min _____

24. mm^3 _____

25. MRI _____

26. NSAID _____

27. $PaCO_2$ _____

28. PaO_2 _____

29. PFT _____

30. pH _____

31. PPD _____

32. PT _____

33. SaO_2 _____

34. TB _____

Exercises and Activities

1. Describe the normal pathway of oxygen through the respiratory system to the bloodstream.

   _____

   _____

   _____

   a. Identify the structures of the respiratory system on the diagram.

alveoli	nasopharynx
diaphragm	respiratory bronchiole
epiglottis	right lower lobe
larynx	right middle lobe
left lower lobe	right upper lobe
left upper lobe	trachea
mainstem bronchus	

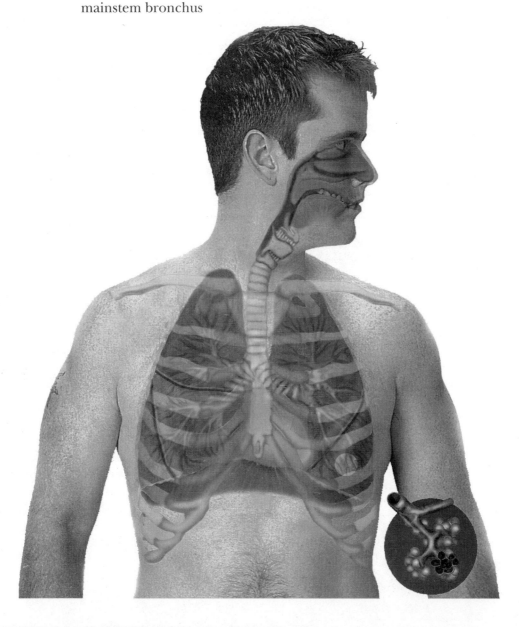

b. Differentiate external respiration and internal respiration.

_____

_____

_____

c. What is the role of surfactant?

_____

_____

d. Differentiate the terms *ventilation* and *perfusion.*

_____

_____

_____

e. What makes us breathe?

_____

_____

2. Describe the items that the nurse would include in a respiratory assessment.

_____

_____

_____

a. Write four questions that the nurse might ask clients about their health history.

(1) _____

(2) _____

(3) _____

(4) _____

b. Briefly describe each of the normal breath sounds.

Bronchial: _____

_____

Bronchovesicular: _____

_____

Vesicular: _____

_____

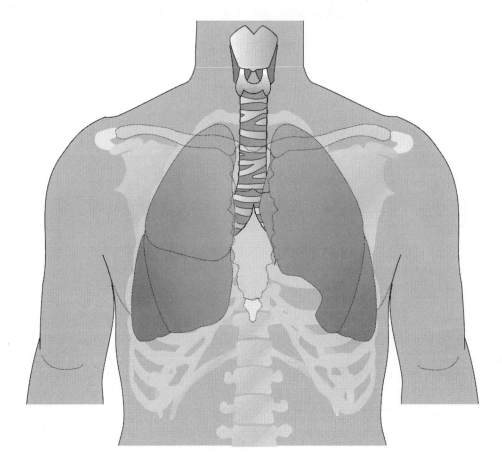

   c. Outline and label on the preceding diagram the areas where you will hear each of the normal breath sounds.

3. What factors are causing an increase in the number of tuberculosis cases in the United States?

_____

_____

_____

   a. Describe the medication and treatment for tuberculosis today.

_____

_____

_____

   b. What factors can contribute to the safety of health care workers exposed to tuberculosis?

_____

_____

_____

4. Compare the following disorders of the respiratory system.

Respiratory Disorder	Risk Factors	Signs and Symptoms	Nursing Interventions
Pneumonia			
Emphysema			
Pulmonary embolus			
Pneumothorax			

5. Janice is a 27-year-old college student in her first semester of nursing classes. She came to the health center today with symptoms of an asthma attack. While giving information for a brief health history, Janice says she's had asthma "all my life" and remembers frequent trips to the clinic and ER as a child. When she was young, dust and pet dander typically triggered her asthma. However, since she moved here from her hometown, Janice feels as if she is having more frequent attacks. Her prescription medication doesn't seem to be as effective. Janice is also worried about her son, Samuel, who may be developing the same problem. Today, she has tightness in her chest and dyspnea. The nurse notes that Janice is leaning forward to breathe, and can hear some wheezing even before using a stethoscope.

   a. List several predisposing factors for asthma.

   _____

   _____

   _____

   b. Describe the changes that are taking place in the airways.

   _____

   _____

   _____

   c. Why is a detailed history important in treating Janice's asthma?

   _____

   _____

   _____

   d. Janice also says she has occasional episodes of bronchitis. How do signs and symptoms of bronchitis differ from those of asthma?

   _____

   _____

   _____

e. List five objective findings that Janice's nurse might detect on assessment today.

(1) _____

(2) _____

(3) _____

(4) _____

(5) _____

f. Describe several nursing interventions that are appropriate for Janice's care.

_____

_____

_____

g. How can client teaching play an important role for Janice and her son?

_____

_____

_____

Self-Assessment Questions

Circle the letter that corresponds to the best answer for each question.

1. While assessing a client's respiratory system, the nurse remembers that a normal finding of the respiratory assessment is
   a. asymmetry of the chest wall and occasional use of the accessory muscles.
   b. bronchial breath sounds over the anterior chest of high pitch and long duration.
   c. vesicular breath sounds over the majority of the lung fields with occasional fine crackles.
   d. bronchovesicular breath sounds by the scapulae posteriorly and near the sternum anteriorly.

2. A client has an increased risk for a pulmonary embolism if she is
   a. on Coumadin therapy.
   b. diabetic or uses OCPs.
   c. between the ages of 20 and 35.
   d. anemic and has episodes of dyspnea.

3. During a physical assessment of the client, the nurse notes Cheyne-Stokes respirations. The description of this respiratory pattern is
   a. irregular periods of increased rate and depth of respiration.
   b. apnea alternating with short periods of shallow respirations.
   c. abnormally slow breathing of increased depth and associated cyanosis.
   d. slow, shallow respirations increasing in rate and depth, alternating with apnea.

4. A nurse is caring for a client with a chest tube in place. If the chest tube is dislodged, the first action of the nurse will be to
   a. evaluate respiratory effort and notify the physician.
   b. replace the tube using sterile gloves and aseptic technique.
   c. cover the opening with petrolatum gauze and apply pressure.
   d. assess the opening on the chest wall for lacerations and drainage.

5. The nurse is examining a client with pneumonia. What abnormal assessment findings are likely to be noted?
   a. Friction rub and stridor
   b. Fine and coarse crackles
   c. Hyperresonance and fever
   e. Bronchovesicular breath sounds

6. The nurse suspects pulmonary edema in a client that has
   a. a chronic cough with purulent sputum.
   b. noticeable wheezing and pain on inspiration.
   c. a cough that produces a large amount of pink, frothy sputum.
   d. absent breath sounds with a mediastinum shift toward the affected side.

Nursing Care of the Client: Cardiovascular System

Key Terms

Match the following terms with their correct definitions.

___ 1. Aneurysm

___ 2. Angina Pectoris

___ 3. Annulus

___ 4. Arteriosclerosis

___ 5. Ascites

___ 6. Atherosclerosis

___ 7. Automatic Implantable Cardioverter-Defibrillator

___ 8. Baseline Level

___ 9. Bradycardia

___10. Cardiac Cycle

___11. Cardiac Output

___12. Cardiac Tamponade

___13. Depolarization

___14. Dyspnea

___15. Dysrhythmia

___16. Embolus

___17. Heart Sound

___18. Hemolysis

___19. Homan's Sign

a. Irregularity in the rate, rhythm, or conduction of the electrical system of the heart.

b. Test to check for the presence of clots in the leg.

c. Inflammation of the myocardium of the heart.

d. Short, high-pitched squeak heard as two inflamed pericardial surfaces rub together.

e. Inflammation in the wall of a vein without clot formation.

f. Treatment that involves injecting a chemical into the vein, causing the vein to become sclerosed (hardened) so blood no longer flows through it.

g. Heart rate in excess of 100 beats per minute in an adult.

h. Formed clot that remains at the site where it formed.

i. Removal of fluid from the pericardial sac.

j. Condition of suddenly awakening, sweating, and having difficulty breathing.

k. Weakness in the wall of a blood vessel.

l. Abnormal accumulation of fluid in the peritoneal cavity.

m. Lab value that serves as a reference point for future value levels.

n. Contraction of the heart.

o. Sound heard by auscultating the heart.

p. Increase in muscle mass.

q. Formation of a clot because of blood pooling in the vessel, trauma to the vessel's endothelial lining, or a coagulation problem with little or no inflammation in the vessel.

r. Inflammation of the membrane sac surrounding the heart.

s. Fluttering or pounding sensation in the chest.

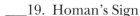

___20. Hypertrophy

    t. Volume of blood pumped by the ventricle with each contraction.

___21. Malignant Hypertension

    u. Formation of a clot due to an inflammation in the wall of the vessel.

___22. Myocardial Infarction

    v. Tissue death as the result of disease or injury.

___23. Myocarditis

    w. Rapidly progressing form of hypertension with the diastolic pressure greater than 120 mm Hg.

___24. Necrosis

    x. Breakdown of red blood cells.

___25. Orthopnea

    y. Difficulty breathing.

___26. Palpitation

    z. Heart rate less than 60 beats per minute in an adult.

___27. Paroxysmal Nocturnal Dyspnea

    aa. Valvular ring in the heart.

___28. Percutaneous Balloon Valvuloplasty

    bb. Insertion of a balloon in a stenosed valve to expand the narrowed valvular space.

___29. Pericardial Friction Rub

    cc. Pressure within a vessel that resists the flow of blood.

___30. Pericardiocentesis

    dd. Inflammation of the skin due to decreased circulation.

___31. Pericarditis

    ee. Surgical removal of a clot.

___32. Peripheral Resistance

    ff. Formation of a clot in a vessel.

___33. Phlebitis

    gg. Tiny metal tube with holes in it that prevents a vessel from collapsing and keeps the atherosclerotic plaque pressed against the vessel wall; any material used to hold tissue in place or provide support.

___34. Phlebothrombosis

    hh. Necrosis (death) of the myocardium caused by an obstruction in a coronary artery.

___35. Primary Hypertension

    ii. Difficulty breathing while lying down.

___36. Repolarization

    jj. Mass, such as a blood clot or an air bubble, that circulates in the bloodstream.

___37. Sclerotherapy

    kk. Volume of blood pumped per minute by the left ventricle.

___38. Secondary Hypertension

    ll. Implantable device that senses a dysrythmia and automatically sends an electrical shock directly to the heart to defibrillate it.

___39. Stasis Dermatitis

    mm. Cardiovascular disease of fatty deposits on the inner lining, the tunica intima, of vessel walls.

___40. Stent

    nn. Narrowing and hardening of arteries.

___41. Stroke Volume

    oo. Chest pain caused by a narrowing of the coronary arteries.

___42. Tachycardia

    pp. Recovery phase of the cardiac muscle.

___43. Thrombectomy

    qq. Diagnostic ultrasonic imaging of the cardiac structures through the esophagus.

___44. Thrombophlebitis

rr. Tying off an involved section of a vein with suture.

___45. Thrombosis

ss. Three factors (pooling of blood, vessel trauma, and a co-agulation problem) that lead to the formation of a clot.

___46. Thrombus

tt. Visibly prominent, dilated, and twisted veins.

___47. Transesophageal Echocardiography

uu. Collection of fluid in the pericardial sac hindering the functioning of the heart.

___48. Varicosities

vv. Introducing a wire into a vein to strip the walls of the vein.

___49. Vasoconstrict

ww. Increase the diameter of a vessel.

___50. Vasodilate

xx. Decrease the diameter of a vessel.

___51. Vein Ligation

yy. Elevated blood pressure greater than 140/90 mm Hg with cause unknown.

___52. Vein Stripping

zz. Elevated blood pressure greater than 140/90 mm. Hg due to another condition within the body.

___53. Virchow's Triad

aaa. Occurs when an electrical impulse transmits completely through the conduction system of the heart and the ventricals contract.

Abbreviation Review

Write the definition of the following abbreviations and acronyms.

1. AAA _____

2. ACE _____

3. AICD _____

4. ALG _____

5. APPT _____

6. AST _____

7. ATG _____

8. AV _____

9. CABG _____

10. CAD _____

11. CAHD _____

12. CBC _____

13. CHF _____

14. CK or CPK _____

15. CPR _____

16. DVT _____

17. EKG _____

18. ESR _____

19. Hct _____

20. HDL _____

21. Hgb _____

22. HTN _____

23. IABP _____

24. ICU _____

25. INR _____

26. LDH _____

27. LDL _____

28. MI _____

29. MRI _____

30. MUGA _____

31. PAC _____

32. PAT _____

33. PSVT _____

34. PT _____

35. PTCA _____

36. PTT _____

37. SA _____

38. SGOT _____

39. TEE _____

40. VAD _____

41. VF _____

42. VLDL _____

43. VT _____

Exercises and Activities

1. Write in the correct terms on the diagram of the heart.

aorta
aortic valve
inferior vena cava
left atrium
left pulmonary artery
left ventricle
mitral valve
pulmonary valve
pulmonary veins
right atrium
right pulmonary artery
right ventricle
superior vena cava
tricuspid valve

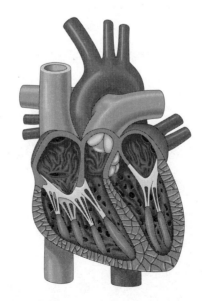

a. Describe the pathway of blood flow through the heart, including the valves (starting with the vena cava).

_____

_____

_____

b. Fill in the blanks with the following terms to describe the electrical pathway of the heart.

atria	Purkinje fibers
atrioventricular (AV) node	QRS complex
bundle branches	right atrium
bundle of His	sinoatrial (SA) node
myocardial cells	ventricles
P wave	

What makes the heart beat? The heart has a conduction system that starts with its own pacemaker. This pacemaker, or the _____, is a small amount of nervous tissue in the _____. From this spot, an electrical impulse spreads across both _____ like "ripples in a pond" and causes them to contract. You can see this on an EKG strip as a _____. The electrical impulse then travels to the _____, where it pauses briefly. This short pause (a tenth of a second) gives the ventricles time to fill with blood. The impulse then proceeds down the AV bundle, which is also called the _____, and continues to the right and left _____. From there, the impulse travels to the _____. These fibers transmit the electrical impulse into the _____, which make the right and left _____ of the heart contract (systole). On an EKG strip, this is seen as the _____.

c. Why are ventricular dysrhythmias more serious than atrial dysrhythmias?

_____

_____

2. What information does the nurse need to obtain from clients about their health history?

_____

_____

_____

a. List five unalterable risk factors for heart disease.

(1) _____

(2) _____

(3) _____

(4) _____

(5) _____

b. How can diet and lifestyle choices modify an individual's risk for heart disease?

_____

_____

c. Why do clients often fail to seek health care for signs and symptoms of cardiac problems?

_____

_____

3. What elements will the nurse include in a thorough assessment of the cardiovascular system?

_____

_____

_____

a. Describe typical symptoms that clients often experience with cardiac disorders.

_____

_____

b. How can clients be assessed for increased fluid volume?

_____

_____

c. Why are breath sounds monitored in clients with cardiac problems?

_____

_____

d. Differentiate findings for arterial occlusion versus venous occlusion in the legs.

_____

_____

_____

4. Describe the following dysrhythmias and discuss their treatment:

	Description	*Treatment*
Atrial fibrillation		
Premature ventricular contractions		
Ventricular tachycardia		
Third degree AV block		

a. List assessment findings and treatment for the following inflammatory disorders:

	Signs/Symptoms	*Treatment*
Infective endocarditis		
Myocarditis		
Mitral valve prolapse		

5. List typical symptoms of a myocardial infarction. How might the symptoms be different for a female client than a male?

a. What is a "silent myocardial infarct"?

b. How does an MI damage the heart?

c. List nursing interventions that will promote recovery for the client following an MI.

d. What client teaching would be needed before discharge?

6. Mr. Williams, a 59-year-old plumber with the city's department of public works, was diagnosed several years ago with primary hypertension. At the time, he was motivated to lose 20 lb, cut back on his smoking, and reduce his stress. However, Mr. Williams eventually became non-compliant when medications that his physician incorporated into his stepped-care treatment plan seemed to cause uncomfortable side effects. Mr. Williams is now admitted to the hospital with congestive heart failure, the result of continued damage from his hypertension.

a. Briefly describe the "stepped-care approach" for management of hypertension.

   b. Why can hypertension lead to congestive heart failure?

   _____

   _____

   c. Name several other conditions that can also result in CHF.

   _____

   _____

   d. If Mr. Williams is diagnosed with left-sided heart failure, what signs and symptoms might be noted on his assessment?

   _____

   _____

   e. List at least five observations that would indicate the right side of his heart is also failing.

   (1) _____

   (2) _____

   (3) _____

   (4) _____

   (5) _____

   f. What medical and nursing interventions will improve Mr. Williams's heart function?

   _____

   _____

   _____

Self-Assessment Questions

Circle the letter that corresponds to the best answer for each question.

1. The cardiac output is equal to the
   a. resting pulse rate for 1 minute.
   b. pulse rate multiplied by the stroke volume.
   c. volume of blood pumped by the left ventricle with each contraction.
   d. volume of blood circulated by the heart in relation to the blood pressure.

2. According to Virchow's triad, the clients most at risk for developing a clot are those with
   a. decreased clotting ability, leg trauma, and obesity.
   b. hypertension, phlebitis, and a positive Homan's sign.
   c. pooling of blood, vessel trauma, and a coagulation problem.
   d. venous stasis, a family history of heart disease, and inactivity.

3. Following a myocardial infarction, your client has started thrombolytic therapy with streptokinase. Which of the following would indicate a serious side effect of this therapy?
   a. Tarry stools
   b. Hypertension
   c. Enlarged lymph nodes
   d. Decreased urine output

4. The first heart sound (S_1) is the sound of the
   a. beginning of diastole.
   b. closing of the mitral and tricuspid valves.
   c. opening of the aortic and pulmonic valves.
   d. closing of the valves on the right side of the heart.

5. Premature ventricular contractions are usually caused by
   a. anxiety.
   b. hypertension.
   c. myocardial ischemia.
   d. coronary artery disease.

6. The nurse is caring for a client who had been on bed rest following surgery. During the assessment, the nurse notes a hardened area in the right calf with warmth and tenderness. The best action for the nurse is to
   a. notify the physician.
   b. gently massage the area to relieve pain.
   c. encourage the client to increase ambulation.
   d. perform and document the Homan's sign for thrombophlebitis.

7. A nurse is caring for a client who has been admitted with CHF. The nurse will administer a vasodilator such as nitroglycerine to this client to
   a. relieve angina.
   b. decrease fluid retention.
   c. improve myocardial contractility.
   d. decrease the amount of blood returning to the heart.

Nursing Care of the Client: Hematologic and Lymphatic Systems

Chapter
20

Key Terms

Match the following terms with their correct definitions.

___ 1. Agranulocytosis

___ 2. Apheresis

___ 3. Bands

___ 4. Blastic Phase

___ 5. Combination Chemotherapy

___ 6. Erythrocytapheresis

___ 7. Fibrinolysis

___ 8. Hemarthrosis

___ 9. Hematocrit

___10. Hematopoiesis

___11. Hemolysis

___12. Hyperuricemia

___13. Idiopathic

___14. Induction Dose

___15. Leukocytosis

___16. Leukopenia

___17. Lymphoma

___18. Maintenance Therapy

___19. Median Survival Time

a. Process of breaking fibrin apart.

b. Intensified phase of leukemia that resembles an acute phase in which there is an increased production of white blood cells.

c. Acute condition causing a severe reduction in the number of granulocytes (basophils, eosinophils, and neutrophils).

d. Decrease in the number of platelets in the blood.

e. Removal of blood from a vein.

f. Increased number of white blood cells.

g. Increased uric acid blood level.

h. Removal of unwanted blood components.

i. Administration of a combination of chemotherapy drugs over a set period of time.

j. Percentage of blood cells in a given volume of blood.

k. Procedure that removes abnormal red blood cells and replaces them with healthy ones.

l. Decreased number of white blood cells.

m. Small doses of chemotherapy given every 3 to 4 weeks to maintain remission.

n. Bleeding into the joints.

o. Increased circulation of immature neutrophils.

p. Process of blood cell production and development.

q. Occurring without a known cause.

r. Immature red blood cell.

s. Condition in which red blood cells become crescent-shaped and elongated.

___20. Microthrombi
___21. Phlebotomy

___22. Purpura
___23. Reticulocyte
___24. Sickled
___25. Thrombocytopenia

t. Average length of life.
u. Reddish-purple patches on the skin indicative of hemorrhage.
v. Tumor of the lymphatic system.
w. Very small clots.
x. Initial dose of chemotherapy.
y. Breakdown of red blood cells.

Abbreviation Review

Write the definition of the following abbreviations and acronyms.

1. ABVD _____
2. ALL _____
3. AML _____
4. ATG _____
5. CHOP _____
6. CLL _____
7. CML _____
8. COPP _____
9. CVP _____
10. DIC _____
11. Hct _____
12. HD _____
13. Hgb _____
14. HLA _____
15. ITP _____
16. LDH _____
17. MOPP _____
18. NHL _____
19. PCA _____
20. PMN _____
21. PT _____
22. PTT _____
23. RBC _____
24. TIBC _____
25. WBC _____

Exercises and Activities

1. What does plasma contain?

_____

a. Identify the following components of blood, giving their purpose and normal laboratory values.

	Purpose	*Normal Values*
RBCs		
WBCs		
Platelets		

b. How do RBCs contribute to oxygenation?

_____

_____

c. Why can reticulocyte counts be used as a diagnostic tool?

_____

_____

2. Label the following diagram of the lymph system.

Axillary node

Cervical node

Inguinal node

Iliac node

Intestinal node

Lymphatic vessel (2)

Palatine tonsil

Peyer's patch

Spleen

Submandibular node

Thymus gland

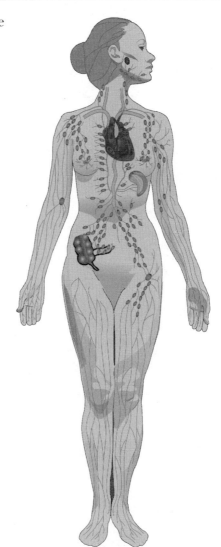

a. Identify the purpose of each of the following:

Lymph nodes: _____

_____

Spleen: _____

_____

Thymus: _____

_____

b. How does the lymphatic system prevent edema?

_____

_____

3. Identify the nursing procedures for administering a blood transfusion.

_____

_____

_____

_____

a. Why can a person with type O negative blood be a universal blood donor?

_____

_____

b. Differentiate among the three types of blood transfusion reactions:
Hemolytic: _____

_____

Febrile: _____

_____

Allergic: _____

_____

c. What is the nurse's responsibility if a blood reaction occurs?

_____

_____

4. Write several questions that you would ask clients about their health history.

(1) _____

(2) _____

(3) _____

(4) _____

(5) _____

(6) _____

(7) _____

(8) _____

  a. What physical findings would be important in assessment of the client?

_____

_____

_____

  b. Briefly describe symptoms and diagnostic tests for the following disorders.

	Symptoms	*Diagnostic Tests*
Iron deficiency anemia		
Polycythemia		
Acute leukemia		
Thrombocytopenia		
Hodgkin's disease		

  c. How would you explain a bone marrow transplant to a client?

_____

_____

  d. What types of clients are at risk for developing DIC?

_____

_____

5. You are caring for Brian, a 23-year-old client who is being evaluated for symptoms of appendicitis, with nausea, vomiting, fever, and abdominal pain. From Brian's health history, you note that he was diagnosed in childhood with hemophilia A, an inherited clotting disorder. Previous laboratory results indicate that his hemophilia is "moderate" and he tends to bleed with surgery or trauma. He is worried that if he needs surgery, it may initiate bleeding for him.

  a. Briefly describe the normal clotting mechanism of the blood. How does hemophilia A interfere with this normal clotting process?

_____

_____

_____

_____

  b. How did Brian acquire this disease?

_____

_____

c. If Brian's hemophilia was severe, what signs and symptoms might he experience?

_____

_____

_____

d. Describe treatment for hemophilia A.

_____

_____

_____

e. If Brian requires surgery for appendicitis, what precautions will be taken? Describe nursing interventions following surgery.

_____

_____

_____

f. What lifestyle precautions should Brian follow at home?

_____

_____

_____

Self-Assessment Questions

Circle the letter that corresponds to the best answer for each question.

1. A client has been diagnosed with thrombocytopenia. The nurse understands that this is a coagulation disorder that includes
   a. a lack of clotting factors in the blood.
   b. microthrombi in arterioles and venules.
   c. a decrease in the number of platelets in the blood.
   d. a syndrome alternating between clotting and hemorrhaging.

2. The nurse is caring for a client with leukemia. The nurse recalls that with this diagnosis, the most likely cause of death will be
   a. DIC.
   b. pneumonia.
   c. heart failure.
   d. hemorrhage.

3. The first sign of Hodgkin's disease in a client is usually
   a. unexplained weight loss.

b. easy bleeding and bruising.

c. painless swelling of a lymph node.

d. tender, enlarged lymph nodes and fever.

4. A nurse is performing an admission assessment on a client with a diagnosis of polycythemia. Which of the following findings would the nurse anticipate when reviewing his laboratory results?

a. High hematocrit

b. Low hemoglobin

c. Low white cell count

d. Increased polymorphs

5. A client has been diagnosed with bacterial sepsis. Because this is a predisposing condition for DIC, the nurse will monitor the client for

a. chills and fever.

b. general fatigue and malaise.

c. swollen and tender lymph nodes.

d. reddish patches on the skin and oozing.

6. Your client is newly diagnosed with Hodgkin's disease. She asks you to tell her about it. You begin by saying that Hodgkin's disease is

a. a rare lymphoma with an unknown cause.

b. a malignancy of the blood-forming tissues.

c. a type of anemia resulting in an increased RBC supply.

d. an inherited hemolytic anemia caused by a recessive gene.

Nursing Care of the Client: Integumentary System

Key Terms

Match the following terms with their correct definitions.

___ 1. Alopecia

___ 2. Angiogenesis

___ 3. Angioma

___ 4. Blanching

___ 5. Cyanosis

___ 6. Debride

___ 7. Ecchymosis

___ 8. Erythema

___ 9. Eschar

___10. Friction

___11. Granulation Tissue

___12. Hemorrhagic Exudate

___13. Hemostasis

___14. Hyperthermia

___15. Hypothermia

___16. Inflammation

___17. Ischemia

___18. Jaundice

a. Pigmented areas in the skin; commonly known as birthmarks or moles.

b. Cessation of bleeding.

c. Abnormal paleness of the skin, seen especially in the face, conjunctiva, nail beds, and oral mucous membranes.

d. To remove dead or damaged tissue or foreign material from a wound.

e. Partial or complete baldness or loss of hair.

f. Condition in which the core body temperature rises above 106°F.

g. Pinpoint hemorrhagic spots on the skin.

h. Discharge that is clear with some blood tinge; seen with surgical incisions.

i. Local and temporary decrease in blood supply.

j. Disruption in the integrity of body tissue.

k. Distended sebaceous gland filled with sebum.

l. Body's defensive adaptation to tissue injury; involves both vascular and cellular responses.

m. Large, irregular hemorrhagic area on the skin; also called a bruise.

n. Formation of new blood vessels.

o. Bluish discoloration of the skin and mucous membranes observed in lips, nail beds, and earlobes.

p. Abnormal growth of scar tissue that is elevated, rounded, and firm with irregular, clawlike margins.

q. Permanent dilation of groups of superficial capillaries and venules; commonly known as "spider veins."

r. Yellowing of the skin, mucous membranes, and sclera of the eyes.

___19. Keloid

s. Force of two surfaces moving against one another.

___20. Keratin

t. Benign vascular tumor involving skin and subcutaneous tissue.

___21. Lipoma

u. White color of the skin when pressure is applied.

___22. Melanin

v. Reddish hue to the skin that may be caused by inflammation of tissues or by sunburn.

___23. Nevi (Nevus)

w. A condition in which the core body temperature drops below 95°F.

___24. Pallor

x. Tough, fibrous protein produced by cells in the epidermis called keratinocytes.

___25. Petechiae

y. Discharge that occurs with severe inflammation accompanied by infection; also called pus.

___26. Purulent Exudate

z. Depigmentation of the skin caused by destruction of melanocytes; appears as milk-white patches on the skin.

___27. Sebaceous Cyst

aa. Oily substance secreted by the sebaceous glands of the skin.

___28. Sebum

bb. Benign tumor consisting of mature fat cells.

___29. Serosanguineous Exudate

cc. Dry, dark, leathery scab composed of denatured protein.

___30. Serous Exudate

dd. Discharge that has a large component of red blood cells.

___31. Shearing

ee. Pigment that gives skin its color.

___32. Telangiectasia

ff. Discharge composed primarily of serum; is watery in appearance and has low protein level.

___33. Vitiligo

gg. Delicate connective tissue consisting of fibroblasts, collagen, and capillaries.

___34. Wound

hh. Force exerted against the skin by movement or repositioning.

Abbreviation Review

Write the definition of the following abbreviations and acronyms.

1. ABCD _____

2. AGF _____

3. FAF _____

4. MRSA _____

5. NPUAP _____

6. PUVA _____

7. ROM _____

8. SPF _____

9. USDHHS _____

10. VAC _____

Exercises and Activities

1. Why is healthy, intact skin important for an individual?

   _____

   _____

   _____

   a. On the following diagram, identify the three layers of the skin and label at least two structures in each layer.

   b. You are caring for a 25-year-old client and a 72-year-old. How would you expect the skin, hair, and nails of your older client to differ from your younger client?

   Skin: _____

   _____

   Hair: _____

   _____

   Nails: _____

   _____

2. A client tells you that she has noticed several small blisters on her left side that are painful. List several questions that you will ask her to gather information about this problem.

   (1) _____

   (2) _____

   (3) _____

   (4) _____

   (5) _____

   (6) _____

(7) _____

(8) _____

a. Identify the seven parameters assessed during the physical examination of the skin. Write two abnormal findings for each parameter.

(1) _____

(2) _____

(3) _____

(4) _____

(5) _____

(6) _____

(7) _____

b. Think of a client you have cared for recently who had a wound, skin lesion, or pressure sore. Use the following diagram to mark the location of the skin problem. Describe its size, shape, appearance, and any drainage. Was it painful? If so, include the type and severity of any pain.

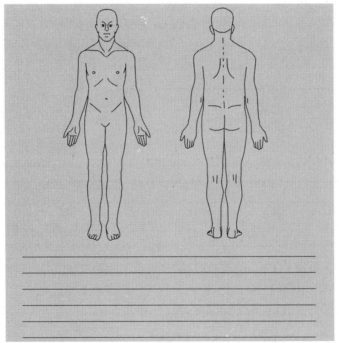

c. Describe the three phases of wound healing. How long does each phase take?

First phase: _____

_____

Second phase: _____

_____

Third phase: _____

_____

d. How does infection slow down the healing process?

_____

_____

_____

3. Two nursing assistants are moving an elderly client up in bed. By sliding the client along the sheets, they cause shearing, which leads to skin breakdown. Why are elderly clients more susceptible to skin breakdown?

_____

_____

_____

a. What is it about moving the client in bed improperly that can cause skin breakdown?

_____

_____

b. What are the risk factors for a pressure ulcer?

_____

_____

c. The next morning, the nurse notices a new reddish patch of skin on the client's sacrum measuring 4 by 6 cm. When the nurse presses on it, the redness doesn't blanch. What has happened?

_____

_____

_____

d. List nursing interventions that can help prevent pressure ulcers.

_____

_____

_____

_____

e. Where are venous stasis ulcers usually found on a client? Draw and label a stasis ulcer on the preceding diagram.

_____

_____

_____

4. List symptoms that a client might experience with the following disorders and at least two nursing/medical interventions for each.

	Symptoms	*Medical/Nursing Interventions*
Carbuncle		
Herpes zoster (shingles)		
Scabies		
Psoriasis		

a. What is the significance of a fourth-degree burn?

_____

_____

_____

b. Identify the goals of treatment after the client with extensive burns is stabilized.

_____

_____

_____

c. What factors make good nutrition difficult for the burn victim?

_____

_____

_____

_____

_____

5. Identify each of these commonly used words by the correct medical term.

Mole _____

Bed sore _____

Birthmarks _____

Athlete's foot _____

Cold sore _____

Shingles _____

Pus _____

6. Lindsey Norton, a 27-year-old client, was in her usual state of good health until 3 days ago when her husband noticed a lesion on her right shoulder. She remembers having a mole

there but says it is now bigger and looks darker. Her skin is very fair, and although she doesn't tan well, she has always loved being in the sun. In fact, she earned money for 2 years in college as a lifeguard. The nurse describes the lesion as having a smooth surface, elevated, with an irregular border, 6 mm in diameter, and bluish-gray in color.

a. Using the examples of skin lesions in your text, what type of lesion might this be?

_____

b. What are the ABCDs of skin cancer?

A: _____

B: _____

C: _____

D: _____

c. Identify risk factors for skin cancer.

_____

_____

d. Lindsey may have malignant melanoma. What medical-surgical interventions would be used for this disease?

_____

_____

_____

e. After Lindsey has the lesion removed, she asks you if she can get skin cancer again. What will you tell her?

_____

_____

_____

f. On the older adult client, where are skin cancers often found?

_____

_____

_____

Self-Assessment Questions

Circle the letter that corresponds to the best answer for each question.

1. The nurse is performing a visual inspection of the skin on a client with psoriasis. With this skin disorder, the nurse would most likely note
   a. red patches covered with thick silvery scales.
   b. large round lesions with a pale center that itch.
   c. painful red lesions with blisters around the trunk.
   d. clusters of vesicles in a linear pattern on the extremities.

2. While assessing the skin of an elderly client, you note an increased number of melanocytes on the face of the client. You recognize that this is a
   a. precursor for melanoma.
   b. normal finding in an older adult.
   c. local reaction to topical creams and ointments.
   d. result of a disease process causing a loss of subcutaneous tissue.

3. The nurse is informing clients about the risk factors for skin cancer. The nurse explains that the major risk factor for skin cancer is
   a. exposure to the sun.
   b. genetic predisposition.
   c. previous radiation therapy.
   d. not using an adequate sun screen lotion.

4. A nursing student is caring for a client with AIDS who has developed mycosis fungoides, a type of malignant disease with skin manifestations. The instructor tells the student that the skin lesions with this disease are
   a. treated with surgical removal and radiation.
   b. caused by a fungus that destroys the epidermis.
   c. similar in appearance to psoriasis in the early stages.
   d. an inflammatory condition of the epidermal and dermal skin layers.

5. A student is preparing to care for a client with third-degree burns on the thorax and arms. The student nurse recalls that third-degree burns
   a. will develop eschar within 2 to 3 days.
   b. are more painful than second-degree burns.
   c. are often associated with muscle and bone damage.
   d. damage the epidermis and dermis and are partial thickness.

6. You are performing a physical assessment on a newly admitted client. You pinch up a fold of skin on your client and observe how quickly and easily it returns to its normal position. This assesses for
   a. moisture.
   b. skin integrity.
   c. skin sensation.
   d. hydration status.

7. A client has third-degree burns resulting from an industrial explosion. After the initial period of stabilization, the most serious complication will be
   a. pain.
   b. scarring.
   c. infection.
   d. respiratory depression.

Nursing Care of the Client: Immune System

Key Terms

Match the following terms with their correct definitions.

___ 1. Allergen

___ 2. Anaphylaxis

___ 3. Angioedema

___ 4. Antibodies

___ 5. Antigen

___ 6. Autoimmune Disorder

___ 7. Autologous

___ 8. Cellular Immunity

___ 9. Diplopia

___10. Exacerbation

___11. Histamine

___12. Homologous

___13. Human Leukocyte Antigen

___14. Humoral Immunity

___15. Hypersensitivity

___16. Immune Response

___17. Immunity

___18. Immunotherapy

___19. Myasthenia Gravis

a. Type of acquired immunity involving T-cell lymphocytes.

b. Excessive reaction to a stimulus.

c. Disease wherein the body identifies its own cells as foreign and activates mechanisms to destroy them.

d. Type of antigen commonly found in the environment.

e. Body's ability to protect itself from foreign agents or organisms.

f. Drooping upper eyelid.

g. A type I systemic reaction to allergens.

h. From the same organism (person).

i. Substance released during allergic reactions.

j. Body's reaction to substances identified as nonself.

k. Decrease or absence of symptoms of a disease.

l. Allergic reaction causing raised pruritic, red, non-tender wheals on the skin; also called hives.

m. Treatment to suppress or enhance immunological functioning.

n. Allergic reaction consisting of edema of subcutaneous layers and mucous membranes.

o. Double vision.

p. Proteins that react with antigens to neutralize or destroy them.

q. Type of immunity dominated by antibodies.

r. Chronic, systemic autoimmune disease characterized by joint stiffness.

s. Autoimmune disease characterized by extreme muscle weakness and fatigue due to the body's inability to transmit nerve impulses to voluntary muscles.

___20. Ptosis
    t. Chronic, progressive, incurable autoimmune disease affecting multiple body organs.

___21. Remission
    u. Any substance identified by the body as nonself.

___22. Rheumatoid Arthritis
    v. Increase in the symptoms of a disease.

___23. Systemic Lupus Erythematosus.
    w. From the same species.

___24. Urticari
    x. Antigen present in human blood.

Abbreviation Review

Write the definition of the following abbreviations and acronyms.

1. ACR _____
2. ANA _____
3. CT _____
4. DMARD _____
5. DNA _____
6. ELISA _____
7. EMG _____
8. ESR _____
9. FDA _____
10. GI _____
11. IgG _____
12. IgM _____
13. LE _____
14. MG _____
15. NIAID _____
16. NPO _____
17. NRTI _____
18. RA _____
19. RF _____
20. ROM _____
21. SLE _____
22. SPF _____

Exercises and Activities

1. How does our immune system protect us against foreign agents or organisms?

_____

_____

_____

a. Compare active and passive acquired immunity and give two examples of each.

_____

_____

_____

b. What factors could depress an individual's immune response?

_____

_____

_____

c. List several symptoms that a client may experience with an immune system disorder.

(1) _____

(2) _____

(3) _____

(4) _____

(5) _____

(6) _____

d. Identify several physical assessment findings that the nurse would note during physical examination of the client.

(1) _____

(2) _____

(3) _____

(4) _____

(5) _____

(6) _____

(7) _____

(8) _____

2. Briefly describe the cause of each type of allergic reaction.

Type I: _____

_____

_____

Type II: _____

_____

_____

Type III: _____

_____

_____

Type IV: _____

_____

_____

a. Circle the three examples of Type I allergic reactions in the following list.

Transfusion reaction	Poison ivy contact dermatitis
Food allergy	Hay fever
Transplant rejection	Anaphylaxis

b. Describe the signs and symptoms of an anaphylactic reaction.

_____

_____

_____

c. What nursing interventions are appropriate for a client with anaphylaxis?

_____

_____

_____

3. Compare the typical manifestations and treatment for each of the following immunological disorders.

	Manifestations	*Treatment/Intervention*
Systemic lupus erythematosus		
Myasthenia gravis		

a. What lifestyle modifications might you recommend for a client with SLE?

_____

_____

_____

4. Ann Lewis, a 34-year-old artist, has been having increasing pain in her hands and knees for some time now. Mornings are really the worst for her, and some days the pain has made it difficult to work. She thought maybe she had a little osteoarthritis like her mother, but Ann's symptoms seem different. At first, her fingers hurt, but now it has spread to her wrists and knees. She has also noticed some nodules on her elbows. During an assessment, you note that her hands feel warm and are showing characteristic signs of rheumatoid arthritis.

a. What triggers the onset of rheumatoid arthritis in an individual?

_____

_____

b. What other symptoms might Ann experience?

_____

_____

c. List signs of rheumatoid arthritis that would be noted during an assessment.

_____

_____

d. Ann tells you she can't quit working, but sometimes her hands are stiff and painful. She's ready to try anything that might help. What medications might be used to control her disease and symptoms?

_____

_____

e. List three goals for this client.
   (1) _____
   (2) _____
   (3) _____

f. What will you advise Ann about her diet and activity?

_____

_____

_____

_____

_____

_____

_____

Self-Assessment Questions

Circle the letter that corresponds to the best answer for each question.

1. The nurse is doing client teaching with a client who has had a severe allergic reaction to a substance. The nurse will emphasize to the client that because of this reaction, it is most important for the client to
   a. wear a Medic Alert tag.
   b. get tested for environmental allergies.
   c. know the signs and symptoms of anaphylaxis.
   d. avoid all situations in which the offending substance might be present.

2. A nurse is performing a physical assessment on a 27-year-old female client admitted with a diagnosis of systemic lupus erythematosus. Which of the following manifestations would the nurse anticipate?
   a. Muscle weakness and fatigue
   b. Fatigue, weight loss, and anemia
   c. Facial rash and painful, swollen joints
   d. Movable, subcutaneous skin nodules

3. A client who received penicillin has developed flushing, facial swelling, and dyspnea. The first intervention will be to administer
   a. epinephrine.
   b. corticosteroids.
   c. an antihistamine.
   d. a different antibiotic.

4. A nurse is caring for a 35-year-old client diagnosed with rheumatoid arthritis. The nurse explains to the client that she may experience periods of remission in the disease alternating with periods of
   a. sensitization.
   b. exacerbation.
   c. susceptibility.
   d. inflammation.

5. A client has received a transplanted kidney. To minimize transplant rejection, this client is most likely to be
   a. given antibiotics prophylactically.
   b. placed in reverse isolation for 2 weeks.
   c. placed on immunosuppressive medications.
   d. monitored for weight loss, fever, and swelling and redness at the transplant site.

Nursing Care of the Client: HIV and AIDS

Key Terms

Match the following terms with their correct definitions.

___ 1. Acquired Immunodeficiency Syndrome

___ 2. Cytomegalovirus

___ 3. Enzyme-Linked Immunosorbent Assay

___ 4. HIV-Wasting Syndrome

___ 5. Human Immunodeficiency Virus

___ 6. Kaposi's Sarcoma

___ 7. *Mycobacterium Avium* Complex

___ 8. Opportunistic Infection

___ 9. *Pneumocystis Carinii* Pneumonia

___10. Seroconversion

___11. Viral Load Test

___12. Western Blot Test

a. Vascular malignancy that can occur any place in the body, including internal organs.

b. Progressively fatal disease that destroys the immune system and the body's ability to fight infection; caused by the human immunodeficiency virus (HIV).

c. Test that measures copies of HIV RNA.

d. The most common opportunistic infection associated with advanced HIV.

e. Basic screening test currently used to detect antibodies to HIV.

f. Unexplained weight loss of more than 10% of body weight accompanied by weakness, chronic diarrhea, and fever in those infected with HIV

g. Confirmatory test used to detect HIV infection.

h. Retrovirus that causes AIDS.

i. Two closely related mycobacteria, *Mycobacterium avium* and *Mycobacterium intracellulare,* that are grouped together.

j. Infection in persons with a defective immune system that rarely causes harm in healthy individuals.

k. Evidence of antibody formation in response to disease or vaccine.

l. One of the herpes type viruses that inhabits saliva, urine, blood, semen, and vaginal secretions.

Abbreviation Review

Write the definition of the following abbreviations and acronyms.

1. ADC _____
2. AFB _____
3. CDC _____
4. CIN _____
5. CMV _____
6. CNS _____
7. ELISA _____
8. HBV _____
9. HCV _____
10. HDV _____
11. HIV _____
12. KS _____
13. MAC _____
14. MDR-TB _____
15. NHL _____
16. NIH _____
17. NNRTI _____
18. OHL _____
19. OSHA _____
20. PCP _____
21. PCR _____
22. PPD _____
23. prn _____
24. RNA _____

Exercises and Activities

1. How is HIV/AIDS diagnosed in a client?

   _____

   _____

   _____

   a. Describe disease progression, from a client's exposure to HIV until AIDS is diagnosed.

   _____

   _____

   _____

b. How does the viral load test help to monitor the status of the client?

_____

_____

_____

2. What are the modes of transmission for HIV infection?

_____

_____

_____

a. Identify risk behaviors associated with HIV infection.

_____

_____

_____

b. What are the trends in HIV/AIDS disease in the United States?

_____

_____

_____

c. A friend confides that she may have been exposed to HIV but is afraid to go for testing. How would you address her fears?

_____

_____

_____

3. Identify several signs and symptoms that might be noted in the initial stages of HIV infection.

(1) _____   (5) _____

(2) _____   (6) _____

(3) _____   (7) _____

(4) _____   (8) _____

a. Why are clients with HIV at risk of developing opportunistic infections?

_____

_____

_____

b. List several opportunistic infections that are often noted in clients with HIV/AIDS.

(1) _____   (6) _____

(2) _____   (7) _____

(3) _____   (8) _____

(4) _____   (9) _____

(5) _____   (10) _____

c. Compare the typical manifestations and treatment for each of the following opportunistic infections or malignancies.

	Manifestations	Treatment/Intervention
Toxoplasmosis		
Kaposi's sarcoma		
CIN		

d. Describe signs and symptoms of HIV-wasting syndrome. How are symptoms controlled?

_____

_____

_____

4. William is a 31-year-old client recently admitted to your medical unit. He acquired HIV disease seven years ago during a homosexual relationship. Following an episode of PCP, he was prescribed secondary prophylaxis, but has been unreliable in taking the medication. On this admission, William has a fever, productive cough, pain in his chest, and malaise. He states that he is also having frequent bouts of diarrhea, which just started again. He had been working on a cleaning crew at night, but is finding it difficult to work because of extreme fatigue. William's physician has ordered tests to rule out TB.

a. Identify tests that would be used to determine if your client has tuberculosis. What results would indicate exposure or active infection?

_____

_____

_____

b. How might symptoms of PCP differ from tuberculosis?

_____

_____

_____

c. What information will you collect during your assessment?

_____

_____

_____

d. Since test results indicate that William has tuberculosis, it is important that he follow treatment guidelines carefully. How will you explain his treatment to him?

_____

_____

_____

e. List several nursing goals for this client.

(1) _____

(2) _____

(3) _____

(4) _____

(5) _____

f. How will you incorporate Standard Precautions when caring for William? Include Airborne and Contact Precautions in your answer.

_____

_____

_____

g. Are there measures William could use to improve his overall health?

_____

_____

_____

Self-Assessment Questions

Circle the letter that corresponds to the best answer for each question.

1. A client is diagnosed with "AIDS" when their CD4 T-cell count is less than 200 cells/mm³ and the client has
   a. at least one opportunistic infection.
   b. a positive Western blot or ELISA test.
   c. symptoms of early HIV disease lasting at least 2 weeks.
   d. a positive viral load test of greater than 200 copies/mL.

2. Which of the following assessments would the nurse expect to observe in the client with histoplasmosis?
   a. abdominal pain and diarrhea
   b. fever, unexplained cough, and malaise
   c. aphthous ulcers, dysphagia, and weight loss
   d. nonproductive cough, night sweats, and fever

3. The nurse explains to the student that the primary goal of medical care for the client diagnosed with HIV is to
   a. prevent the spread of HIV to others.
   b. detect progression to AIDS as early as possible.
   c. keep the disease from progressing as long as possible.
   d. maintain the comfort of the client with symptoms of opportunistic infections.

4. The primary modes of transmission for HIV infection include all but which of the following?
   a. urine
   b. blood
   c. amniotic fluid
   d. vaginal secretions

5. The nurse knows that the development of nutritional malabsorption in the client with HIV-Wasting Syndrome is most directly the result of
    a. side effects of HIV/AIDS medications.
    b. aphthous ulcers of the mouth and esophagus.
    c. food intolerances related to change in taste perception.
    e. injury to the small intestine by opportunistic infections.

Nursing Care of the Client: Musculoskeletal System

Key Terms

Match the following terms with their correct definitions.

___ 1. Amphiarthrosis

___ 2. Amputation

___ 3. Arthroplasty

___ 4. Bruxism

___ 5. Closed Reduction

___ 6. Contracture

___ 7. Crepitus

___ 8. Diarthrosis

___ 9. Dislocation

___10. Fracture

___11. Heberden's Nodes

___12. Kyphosis

___13. Locomotor

___14. Lordosis

___15. Open Reduction

___16. Orthopedics (Orthopaedics)

___17. Osteoporosis

___18. Paresthesia

___19. Phantom Limb Pain

a. Repair of a fracture done without surgical intervention.

b. Condition characterized by slightly movable joints such as the vertebrae.

c. Injury in which the articular surfaces of a joint are no longer in contact.

d. Pertaining to movement or the ability to move.

e. Branch of medicine that deals with the prevention or correction of the disorders and diseases of the musculoskeletal system.

f. Cutting a hole in a plaster cast to relieve pressure on the skin or a bony area and to permit visualization of the underlying body part.

g. Lateral curvature of the spine.

h. Surgical procedure that enables the surgeon to reduce (repair) a fracture under direct visualization.

i. Replacement of both articular surfaces within a joint capsule.

j. Grating or crackling sensation or sound.

k. Increased roundness of the thoracic spinal curve.

l. Abnormal sensation such as numbness or tingling.

m. Immovable joint.

n. Exaggeration of the curvature of the lumbar spine.

o. Freely movable joint.

p. Subcutaneous nodules of sodium urate crystals.

q. Teeth grinding during sleep.

r. Break in the continuity of a bone.

s. Sensation of pain, soreness, and stiffness in an amputated limb.

___20. Scoliosis

t. Injury to ligaments surrounding a joint caused by a sudden twist, wrench, or fall.

___21. Sprain

u. Removal of all or part of an extremity.

___22. Strain

v. Permanent shortening of a muscle.

___23. Subluxation

w. Enlargement and characteristic hypertrophic spurs in the terminal interphalangeal finger joints.

___24. Synarthrosis

x. Increase in the porosity of bone.

___25. Tophi

y. Injury to a muscle or tendon due to overuse or over-stretching.

___26. Windowing

z. Partial separation of an articular surface.

Abbreviation Review

Write the definition of the following abbreviations and acronyms.

1. BMD _____

2. CMS _____

3. CPM _____

4. DJD _____

5. NIAMS _____

6. NOF _____

7. ORIF _____

8. RICE _____

9. ROM _____

10. SCD _____

11. TMJ _____

Exercises and Activities

1. Label each of the bones on this diagram.

Clavicle
Cranium
Femur
Fibula
Humerus
Maleolus
Mandible
Patella
Pelvis
Phalanges
Radius
Rib
Sternum
Tibia
Ulna
Vertebral column
Scapula

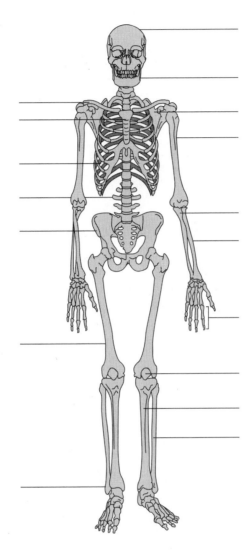

a. Draw a line from each type of diarthrosis joint to a place where it is found on the skeleton.
   Hinge
   Pivot
   Gliding
   Ball and socket
   Saddle

b. What is the difference between voluntary and involuntary muscle?

_____

_____

_____

c. Identify these spinal curvatures.

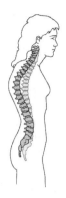

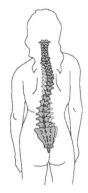

_____   _____

The type of curvature seen in pregnancy is _____.

The type of curvature associated with osteoporosis is _____.

Adolescents are assessed for a curvature called _____.

2. What is included in an assessment of the musculoskeletal system?

_____

_____

_____

_____

a. List several assessment findings that would be abnormal for a joint.

_____

_____

_____

b. How could you assess for ROM:

For the neck? _____

_____

For the hip? _____

_____

c. Why is an assessment made of the client's ability to perform ADLs?

_____

_____

_____

3. Name and describe the types of fractures pictured here.

a. _____

_____

_____

_____

_____

_____

b. _____

_____

_____

_____

_____

_____

c. Your client had a long arm cast applied 1 hour ago. How will you assess the cast?

_____

_____

_____

List the "five Ps" for the neurovascular assessment of this client.

(1) _____

(2) _____

(3) _____

(4) _____

(5) _____

How often will you assess the client?

_____

_____

d. Describe the signs and symptoms of three complications of a fracture.

Infection: _____

_____

Fat embolism: _____

_____

Compartment syndrome: _____

_____

c. List three types of traction. Describe nursing care for a client in traction.

_____

_____

_____

4. Identify ten risk factors for osteoporosis.

(1) _____   (6) _____

(2) _____   (7) _____

(3) _____   (8) _____

(4) _____   (9) _____

(5) _____   (10) _____

a. Why are individuals with osteoporosis more likely to suffer fractures?

_____

_____

b. What will you include in your teaching (diet, activity, safety) for a client who is newly diagnosed with osteoporosis?

_____

_____

_____

_____

5. Mrs. Castro, a 61-year-old client, has been diagnosed with degenerative joint disease (osteoarthritis). Although she used to be quite active with her family and her favorite hobby, which was gardening, she now has problems with stiffness and pain in her knees, especially on her right side. An old injury to her right knee many years ago is probably contributing to the additional pain and loss of mobility on that side now. Mrs. Castro acknowledges that she needs to lose some of her extra weight and at first attributed her knee problems to "old age." She asks you for more information about this disorder.

a. Describe the signs and symptoms of degenerative joint disease.

_____

_____

_____

b. How will you explain the changes that are occurring in DJD?

_____

_____

_____

c. What type of lifestyle changes and medication might be suggested for Mrs. Castro?

_____

_____

_____

d. The next time you see Mrs. Castro, she admits she has lost only a few pounds but has been trying medication and uses a cane for support. Now, however, she can hardly climb the stairs in her house and is in almost constant pain. Mrs. Castro is scheduled for arthroplasty on her right knee. Briefly describe this surgery.

_____

_____

_____

e. What nursing care and interventions will be needed following total knee replacement?

_____

_____

_____

f. What are your goals for this client?

_____

_____

_____

_____

_____

Self-Assessment Questions

Circle the letter that corresponds to the best answer for each question.

1. The nurse is caring for a client following surgery on the right leg. Because the physician's order is for the client to use a three-point gait, the nurse will instruct the client to move
   a. both crutches with the right leg, then move the left leg.
   b. both crutches, then move both legs by swinging them through.
   c. the right leg with the left crutch, then the left leg with the right crutch.
   d. the right crutch, then the left foot, then the left crutch, then the right foot.

2. A client has recently had a cast applied to the arm. When the nurse assesses this client, which of the following findings would be considered abnormal?
   a. There is a capillary refill of almost 2 seconds in the fingers.
   b. The cast is cool to the touch and sounds dull when percussed.
   c. The client is experiencing pain that is relieved with analgesics.
   d. The client reports a tingling sensation relieved with position change.

3. A client has been recently diagnosed with osteoporosis. When giving discharge instructions to the client, the nurse will include all but which of the following suggestions?
   a. Reduce caffeine intake.
   b. Increase protein intake.
   c. Increase calcium intake.
   d. Increase weight-bearing activity.

4. Your client mentions that she used to sew children's clothing several hours a week until she started experiencing burning and numbness in her thumb and fingers, particularly in her right hand. You recall that these are most likely subjective findings for
   a. bursitis.
   b. osteoarthritis.
   c. rheumatoid arthritis.
   d. carpal tunnel syndrome.

5. The nurse is caring for a client who has had a cast applied following a fracture. To complete a neurovascular assessment on the client, the nurse will assess every 15 to 30 minutes for
   a. edema and joint mobility.
   b. drainage and temperature.
   c. pain, edema, and capillary return.
   d. pallor, paresthesia, and level of consciousness.

6. A client is admitted with osteomyelitis in an extremity. When reviewing the care of this client with the nursing assistant, the nurse emphasizes the need to
   a. keep the extremity at complete rest.
   b. elevate the extremity to decrease edema.
   c. begin passive ROM exercises to the extremity.
   d. gently massage the extremity to increase circulation.

Nursing Care of the Client: Neurological System

Key Terms

Match the following terms with their correct definitions.

___ 1. Affect

    a. Peculiar sensation preceding a seizure or migraine; may be a taste, smell, sight, sound, dizziness, or just a "funny feeling."

___ 2. Agnosia

    b. Inflammation of the meninges.

___ 3. Anosognosia

    c. Paralysis of lower extremities.

___ 4. Aphasia

    d. Difficulty in swallowing.

___ 5. Areflexia

    e. That part of the peripheral nervous system consisting of the sympathetic and parasympathetic nervous systems and controlling unconscious activities.

___ 6. Ataxia

    f. Inability to recognize, either by sight or sound, familiar objects, such as a hand.

___ 7. Aura

    g. Cessation of motor, sensory, autonomic, and reflex impulses below the level of injury; characterized by flaccid paralysis of all skeletal muscles, loss of spinal reflexes, loss of sensation, and absence of autonomic function below the level of injury.

___ 8. Automatism

    h. Person's ability to perceive environmental stimuli and body reactions and then to respond with thought and action.

___ 9. Autonomic Nervous System

    i. System of the brain and spinal cord.

___10. Bradykinesia

    j. Acute, prolonged episode of seizure activity that lasts at least 30 minutes and may or may not involve loss of consciousness.

___11. Central Nervous System

    k. Lack of awareness regarding deficits.

___12. Cephalalgia

    l. Weakness of one side of the body.

___13. Chorea

    m. Ability to recognize an object by feel.

___14. Dysarthria

    n. Pain and rigidity in the neck.

___15. Dysphagia

    o. Nerves that connect the central nervous system to the skin and skeletal muscles and control conscious activities.

___16. Emotional Lability

    p. Headache; also known as cephalgia.

___17. Encephalitis

q. Inability to communicate; often the result of a brain lesion.

___18. Fasciculation

r. Slowness of voluntary movement and speech.

___19. Glasgow Coma Scale

s. Dizziness.

___20. Graphesthesia

t. Hardened tissue.

___21. Hemiparesis

u. Failure to recognize or care for one side of the body.

___22. Hemiplegia

v. Objective tool for assessing consciousness in clients with head injuries.

___23. Homonymous Hemianopia

w. Difficult and defective speech due to a dysfunction of the muscles used for speech.

___24. Kernig's Sign

x. Loss of vision in half of the visual field on the same side of both eyes.

___25. Meningitis

y. Constant, involuntary movement of the eye in various directions.

___26. Mentation

z. Outward expression of mood or emotion.

___27. Neuralgia

aa. Inability to coordinate voluntary muscle action.

___28. Neurogenic Shock

bb. Diagnostic test for inflammation in the nerve roots; the inability to extend the leg when the thigh is flexed against the abdomen.

___29. Neurotransmitter

cc. Chemical substance that excites, inhibits, or modifies the response of another neuron.

___30. Nuchal Rigidity

dd. Mechanical, repetitive motor behavior performed unconsciously.

___31. Nystagmus

ee. Loss of emotional control.

___32. Orientation

ff. Dysfunction or paralysis of both arms, both legs, and bowel and bladder.

___33. Paraplegia

gg. Absence of reflexes.

___34. Peripheral Nervous System

hh. Ability to concentrate, remember, or think abstractly.

___35. Quadriplegia

ii. Inflammation of the brain.

___36. Responsiveness

jj. Person's awareness of self in relation to person, place, time, and, in some cases, situation.

___37. Sclerotic

kk. Hypotensive situation resulting from the loss of sympathetic control of vital functions from the brain.

___38. Somatic Nervous System

ll. Involuntary twitching of muscle fibers.

___39. Spinal Shock

mm. System of cranial nerves, spinal nerves, and the autonomic nervous system.

___40. Status Epilepticus

nn. Ability to identify letters, numbers, or shapes drawn on the skin.

___41. Stereognosis

oo. Paralysis of one side of the body.

___42. Unilateral Neglect

    pp. Paroxysmal pain that extends along the course of one or more nerves.

___43. Vertigo

    qq. Condition characterized by abnormal, involuntary, purposeless movements of all musculature of the body.

Abbreviation Review

Write the definition of the following abbreviations and acronyms.

1. ACTH _____
2. AD _____
3. ALS _____
4. ANS _____
5. CN _____
6. CSF _____
7. CT _____
8. CVA _____
9. DAI _____
10. EEG _____
11. GABA _____
12. IgG _____
13. MAO _____
14. MAP _____
15. MS _____
16. MSG _____
17. NSAID _____
18. $PaCO_2$ _____
19. PERRLA _____
20. PNS _____
21. PT _____
22. RIND _____
23. SCI _____
24. TIA _____

Exercises and Activities

1. Identify the following landmarks on the diagram below.

   Broca's area

   Cerebellum

   Diencephalon

   Frontal lobe

   Midbrain

   Medulla oblongata

   Occipital lobe

   Parietal lobe

   Pons

   Spinal cord

   Temporal lobe

   Wernicke's area

   a. Describe the main function for each of the following:

   Spinal nerves _____
   _____

   Cranial nerves _____
   _____

   Somatic nervous system _____
   _____

   Autonomic nervous system _____
   _____

   b. Give the name and one method of assessing for each cranial nerve.

CN	Name	Assessment
I		
II		

CN	Name	Assessment
III		
IV		
V		
VI		
VII		
VIII		
IX, X		
XI		
XII		

2. List the components of a complete nursing assessment of the neurological system.

_____

_____

_____

_____

   a. What observations can be used to assess the client for each of the following items?

Communication _____

Emotional status _____

Intellectual function _____

Mental status _____

Orientation _____

   b. How is the Glasgow Coma Scale used to determine the level of consciousness?

_____

_____

3. What signs and symptoms might be noted in a client with increased intracranial pressure?

_____

_____

   a. List several factors that can cause an increase in intracranial pressure.

     (1) _____

     (2) _____

     (3) _____

     (4) _____

     (5) _____

     (6) _____

b. Briefly describe the medical/surgical treatment that may be used for a client with a head injury.

_____

_____

c. You are asked to perform frequent assessment on the neurological status of your client. What will you include?

_____

_____

_____

4. List several risk factors for stroke. Circle the major risk factor.

(1) _____   (5) _____   (9) _____

(2) _____   (6) _____   (10) _____

(3) _____   (7) _____   (11) _____

(4) _____   (8) _____   (12) _____

a. What intellectual deficits may occur with a stroke?

_____

_____

_____

b. Describe medical/surgical management of the client with a stroke.

_____

_____

_____

_____

c. List several factors that can cause seizures.

(1) _____   (5) _____   (9) _____

(2) _____   (6) _____   (10) _____

(3) _____   (7) _____   (11) _____

(4) _____   (8) _____   (12) _____

d. How would you differentiate among the three types of generalized seizures?

Tonic-clonic (grand mal): _____

_____

Absence (petit mal): _____

_____

Myoclonic: _____

_____

   e. You are helping a client to the bathroom when the client begins to have a tonic-clonic (grand mal) seizure. What actions will you take?

_____

_____

_____

5. What priorities are used when caring for a client in the acute phase of spinal injury?

_____

_____

_____

   a. Identify factors that can cause autonomic dysreflexia in the client with spinal injury.

_____

_____

_____

   b. Describe immediate care of the client experiencing autonomic dysreflexia.

_____

_____

_____

   c. Identify the signs and symptoms and medical treatment for the following neurological disorders.

Disorder	Signs/Symptoms	Treatment
Parkinson's disease		
Amyotrophic lateral sclerosis (ALS)		
Alzheimer's disease		

   d. What are the goals of nursing care in the late stage of Alzheimer's disease? Why is respite care important for family caregivers?

_____

_____

_____

_____

6. Until this year, Mr. Krause, a 32-year-old high school math teacher, was active as the school's soccer coach, lifted weights at the gym, and enjoyed taking his son for bicycle rides. During the last several months, he had noticed occasional weakness in his legs, which he attributed to long hours coaching and perhaps his age. When Mr. Krause started to walk unsteadily and even fall a couple of times, he became increasingly concerned, but hoped it was just fatigue. After an episode of double vision, he agreed to see his physician. Following a thorough health

history and physical examination, multiple sclerosis (MS) was suspected. Several tests were ordered to try to confirm the diagnosis.

a. What tests can be done to help determine if Mr. Krause has MS?

  _____

  _____

b. What other symptoms do clients with MS experience in the early stages of the disease?

  _____

  _____

  _____

c. Mr. Krause asks why his symptoms seem to come and go. How would you describe the disease process to him?

  _____

  _____

  _____

  _____

d. If Mr. Krause has the relapsing-remitting type of MS, what will that mean for his symptoms and prognosis?

  _____

  _____

  _____

e. You are reviewing with Mr. Krause lifestyle changes that may be helpful. What measures can he take to limit exacerbations of his disease?

  _____

  _____

  _____

f. Write three nursing diagnoses or goals for Mr. Krause.

  (1) _____

  (2) _____

  (3) _____

g. Briefly describe medical management of MS.

  _____

  _____

h. How can Mr. Krause maintain his mobility as his disease progresses?

  _____

  _____

i. What safety measures would you include in teaching Mr. Krause and his wife?

  _____

  _____

Self-Assessment Questions

Circle the letter that corresponds to the best answer for each question.

1. During a neurological assessment, a nurse asks the client to explain the meaning of a proverb such as "a stitch in time saves nine." The nurse is assessing the client's
   a. language and recall.
   b. intellectual functioning.
   c. orientation and awareness.
   d. understanding of American culture.

2. Several hours following a head injury, the client's score on the Glasgow Coma Scale changes from 13 to 9. The nurse responds appropriately by
   a. notifying the physician.
   b. reassessing after the client has time to rest.
   c. charting improvement in the client's condition.
   d. continuing to assess at regular intervals, at least every 2 hours.

3. The student nurse is preparing to care for a client with a T-4 spinal injury. The student recalls that this client is at risk of developing autonomic dysreflexia, which can lead to
   a. spinal shock.
   b. cardiac arrest.
   c. a hypertensive crisis.
   d. a loss of respiratory function.

4. The nursing student is caring for a client with a left-sided CVA who is experiencing aphasia. The student anticipates this client will have difficulty with
   a. coordination.
   b. communication.
   c. chewing and swallowing.
   d. recognizing familiar objects.

5. The nurse is discussing self-care measures with the client who takes L-Dopa for Parkinson's disease. The nurse advises the client to
   a. avoid high-protein foods.
   b. take a multivitamin daily.
   c. eat foods high in vitamin B_6.
   d. adjust the dose according to symptoms.

Nursing Care of the Client: Sensory System

Key Terms

Match the following terms with their correct definitions.

___ 1. Acoustic Neuroma

___ 2. Affect

___ 3. Afferent Nerve Pathway

___ 4. Arousal

___ 5. Astigmatism

___ 6. Awareness

___ 7. Cataract

___ 8. Cerumen

___ 9. Chalazion

___10. Cognition

___11. Conductive Hearing Loss

___12. Conjunctivitis

___13. Consciousness

___14. Disorientation

___15. Efferent Nerve Pathway

___16. Glaucoma

___17. Hallucination

___18. Hyperopia

a. Condition in which the lens of the eye loses its transparency and becomes opaque.

b. Expression of mood or feeling.

c. Condition characterized by the inability of the sound waves to reach the inner ear.

d. Ability to evaluate alternatives to arrive at an appropriate course of action.

e. Disorder characterized by an abnormally high pressure of fluid inside the eyeball.

f. Condition in which the inner ear or cochlear portion of cranial nerve VIII is abnormal or diseased.

g. Change in the perception of sensory stimuli; can affect any of the senses.

h. Dizziness.

i. Conductive hearing loss secondary to a pathologic change of the bones in the middle ear.

j. Inflammation of the middle ear.

k. Repetitive and involuntary movement of the eyeballs.

l. Inability of the eyes to focus in the same direction.

m. State of awareness of self, others, and surrounding environment.

n. Inaccurate perception or misinterpretation of sensory stimuli.

o. Sensorineural hearing loss associated with aging.

p. Descending spinal cord pathway that transmits sensory impulses from the brain.

q. Inflammation of the conjunctiva.

r. Asymmetric focus of light rays on the retina.

___19. Illusion

___20. Judgment

___21. Keratitis

___22. Macular Degeneration

___23. Ménière's Disease

___24. Mood

___25. Myopia

___26. Nystagmus

___27. Orientation

___28. Otitis Externa

___29. Otitis Media

___30. Otosclerosis

___31. Perception

___32. Presbycusis

___33. Presbyopia

___34. Sensation

___35. Sensorineural Hearing Loss

___36. Sensory Deficit

___37. Sensory Deprivation

___38. Sensory Overload

___39. Sensory Perception

___40. Strabismus

___41. Stye

s. State of excessive and sustained multisensory stimulation manifested by behavior change and perceptual distortion.

t. Bacterial infection of the external ear canal skin.

u. Intellectual ability to think.

v. Capacity to perceive sensory impressions through thoughts and actions.

w. Nearsightedness.

x. Ability to receive and process stimuli received through the sensory organs.

y. State of mental confusion in which awareness of time, place, self, and/or situation is impaired.

z. Ascending spinal cord pathway that transmits sensory impulses to the brain.

aa. Atrophy or deterioration of the macula.

bb. A sensory perception that occurs in the absence of external stimuli and not based on reality.

cc. Earwax.

dd. Farsightedness.

ee. Perception of self in relation to the surrounding environment.

ff. State of reduced sensory input from the internal or external environment, manifested by alterations in sensory perception.

gg. Ability to receive sensory impressions and, through cortical association, relate the stimuli to past experiences and form an impression of the nature of the stimulus.

hh. State of wakefulness and alertness.

ii. Cyst of the meibomian glands.

jj. State of hearing loss characterized by tinnitus and vertigo.

kk. Ability to experience, recognize, organize, and interpret sensory stimuli.

ll. Inflammation of the cornea.

mm. Inability of the lens of the eye to change curvature to focus on near objects.

nn. Feeling.

oo. Pustular inflammation of an eyelash follicle or sebaceous gland on the eyelid margin.

___42. Tinnitus

pp. Ringing sound in the ear.

___43. Vertigo

qq. Slow-growing, benign tumor of the vestibular portion of the inner ear.

Abbreviation Review

Write the definition of the following acronyms.

1. ANS _____

2. CNS _____

3. IOL _____

4. IOP _____

5. LOC _____

6. PNS _____

7. TDD _____

8. UPSIT _____

Exercises and Activities

1. In what ways is an intact, functioning sensory system important for an individual?

   _____

   _____

   _____

   a. How would you differentiate perception and cognition?

      _____

      _____

   b. Describe aspects of the hospital environment that can distort a client's perception of time.

      _____

      _____

      (1) How can hospitalization contribute to sensory overload?

          _____

          _____

      (2) How can hospitalization contribute to sensory deficit?

          _____

          _____

c. A nursing assistant tells you, "Mrs. Davis doesn't seem to be very alert this morning. I tried to help her eat her breakfast, but she just kept staring, not smiling at me or saying anything. It was like I wasn't even there." List the components of cognition, and circle the ones that are altered in Mrs. Davis today.

(1) _____   (4) _____
(2) _____   (5) _____
(3) _____   (6) _____

d. Write two questions that the nurse could ask a client to determine immediate, recent, and remote memory.

Immediate   (1) _____
             (2) _____
Recent   (1) _____
             (2) _____
Remote   (1) _____
             (2) _____

2. Label the diagram of the eye using the terms listed below.

Anterior chamber

Ciliary body

Conjunctiva

Cornea

Fovea centralis

Iris

Lens

Optic disk

Optic nerve

Posterior chamber

Pupil

Retina

Sclera

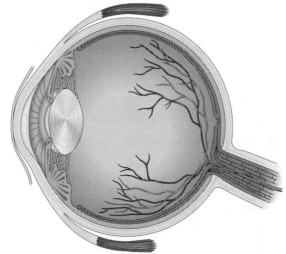

a. Name each structure that light passes through to reach the retina.

_____
_____

b. Identify the structures of the ear on the following diagram. Draw a circle around the middle ear.

Auricle
Cochlea
Cranial nerve VIII
Eustachian tube
External auditory
    canal
Incus
Malleus
Round window
Semicircular canals
Stapes
Tympanic membrane

c. What changes occur in these senses with aging?

Hearing: _____

_____

Vision: _____

_____

Touch: _____

_____

d. Identify each of these common terms by the correct medical term.

Earwax _____

Eardrum _____

Nearsighted _____

Swimmer's ear _____

Dizziness _____

Pinkeye _____

3. What interventions might help a hospitalized client with visual impairment?

_____

_____

_____

a. Identify safety measures for a client with vertigo.

_____

_____

b. Your friend tells you she must be "legally blind" because she can't even see the first letter on the eye chart without her glasses. Is she correct?

_____

_____

c. List symptoms a client would experience with the following disorders and the treatment.

Disorder	Symptoms	Treatment
Ménière's disease		
Retinal detachment		
Glaucoma		
Cataracts		

4. A new client has recently arrived at your long-term care facility for a brief stay following discharge from the hospital. The nursing assistant tells you, "Mr. Döring doesn't do anything I ask. He acts as if he can't hear me."

a. Describe behaviors that might indicate a hearing loss in a client.

_____

_____

_____

b. After reviewing the chart and assessing Mr. Döring, you determine he has a moderate hearing loss and uses a hearing aid, which was left at the hospital. What interventions can help you to communicate with your client for now?

_____

_____

_____

_____

c. During his morning care, the nursing assistant notices that his right eyelid is crusted over and the eye looks reddened. You are concerned that he may have conjunctivitis. What other symptoms might be present? What special precautions will you take?

_____

_____

_____

_____

d. Mr. Döring seems to have a poor appetite. When you ask, he tells you nothing tastes very good. What changes occur in taste and smell with aging? How can these changes cause nutrition problems?

_____

_____

_____

_____

Self-Assessment Questions

Circle the letter that corresponds to the best answer for each question.

1. A nurse caring for a client recovering from surgery notes that he is still very drowsy from medication. This client is exhibiting an alteration in
   a. affect.
   b. arousal.
   c. sensation.
   d. cognition.

2. The nurse is performing a physical assessment on a client with a diagnosis of acoustic neuroma affecting cranial nerves VII and VIII. Which of these findings will the nurse anticipate?
   a. Tinnitus and ear pain
   b. Conductive hearing loss
   c. Facial weakness and vertigo
   d. Loss of hearing and nystagmus

3. You observe your client turning his head to use peripheral vision when talking with you. You recall that this may occur with
   a. cataracts.
   b. presbyopia.
   c. retinal detachment.
   d. macular degeneration.

4. A home health care nurse is providing care for an older adult client. A family member mentions that the client is showing changes in speech patterns and habits. The nurse states that these changes may indicate
   a. hearing loss.
   b. disorientation.
   c. sensory overload.
   d. normal effects of aging.

5. The nurse is admitting a client to a long-term care facility following a stroke. Because the client also has a diagnosis of glaucoma, the physician orders
   a. antibiotics.
   b. mydriatic drops.
   c. topical anesthetic.
   d. pilocarpine drops.

6. Your client, who is newly diagnosed with open-angle glaucoma, asks you why this could cause blindness. You reply that
    a. increased pressure within the eye causes a detachment of the retina.
    b. an increase in fluid in the front of the eye damages the lens, causing loss of vision.
    c. the fluid in the eye puts pressure on the neurons of the retina, which destroys them.
    d. an inflammatory response in the posterior chamber of the eye damages the optic nerve.

Nursing Care of the Client: Endocrine System

Chapter 27

Key Terms

Match the following terms with their correct definitions.

___ 1. Agranulocytosis

___ 2. Autosomal

___ 3. Chvostek's Sign

___ 4. Cretinism

___ 5. Dawn Phenomenon

___ 6. Endocrine

___ 7. Exophthalmos

___ 8. Glucagon

___ 9. Glycosuria

___10. Goiter

___11. Gynecomastia

___12. Hirsutism

___13. Hormone

___14. Hyperglycemia

___15. Hypoglycemia

a. Early morning glucose elevation produced by the release of growth hormone.

b. Marked protrusion of the eyeballs resulting from increased orbital fluid behind the eyeballs.

c. Acute condition causing a severe reduction in the number of granulocytes (basophils, eosinophils, and neutrophils).

d. Substance that initiates or regulates activity of another organ, system, or gland in another part of the body.

e. Hormone secreted by the alpha cells of the pancreas, which stimulates release of glucose by the liver.

f. Low blood glucose.

g. Descriptor for a symptom that begins and ends abruptly.

h. Caused by treatment or diagnostic procedures.

i. Hormone produced and secreted by the beta cells in the islets of Langerhans of the pancreas.

j. Increased urination.

k. Sharp flexion of the wrist and ankle joints, involving muscle twitching or cramps.

l. Abnormal enlargement of one or both breasts in males.

m. Pertaining to a condition transmitted by a nonsex chromosome.

n. Congenital condition due to a lack of thyroid hormones causing defective physical development and mental retardation.

o. Group of cells secreting substances directly into the blood or lymph circulation and affecting another part of the body.

___16. Hypovolemia

___17. Iatrogenic

___18. Insulin

___19. Ketonuria

___20. Lipodystrophy

___21. Myxedema

___22. Paroxysmal

___23. Polydipsia

___24. Polyphagia

___25. Polyuria

___26. Somogyi Phenomenon

___27. Tetany

___28. Trousseau's Sign

p. Excessive body hair in a masculine distribution.

q. Severe hypothyroidism in adults.

r. In response to hypoglycemia, the release of glucose-elevating hormones (epinephrine, cortisol, glucagon), which produces a hyperglycemic state.

s. Carpal spasm caused by inflating a blood pressure cuff above the client's systolic pressure and leaving it in place for 3 minutes.

t. Abnormal spasm of the facial muscles in response to a light tapping of the facial nerve.

u. Presence of excessive glucose in the urine.

v. Elevated blood glucose.

w. Enlargement of the thyroid gland.

x. Increased hunger.

y. Abnormally low circulatory blood volume.

z. Presence of ketones (acidic by-products of fat metabolism) in the urine.

aa. Excessive thirst.

bb. Atrophy or hypertrophy of subcutaneous fat.

Abbreviation Review

Write the meaning or definition of the following abbreviations and acronyms.

1. ACTH _____

2. ADA _____

3. ADH _____

4. CDC _____

5. CVA _____

6. DKA _____

7. EKG _____

8. FSH _____

9. GDM _____

10. GH _____

11. HHNK _____

12. IDDM _____

13. IGT _____

14. IV _____

15. LH _____

16. MSH _____

17. NIDDM _____

18. PTH _____

19. PTU _____

20. PVD _____

21. TSH _____

Exercises and Activities

1. Write the name of each unidentified endocrine gland in the diagram and at least one of its functions.

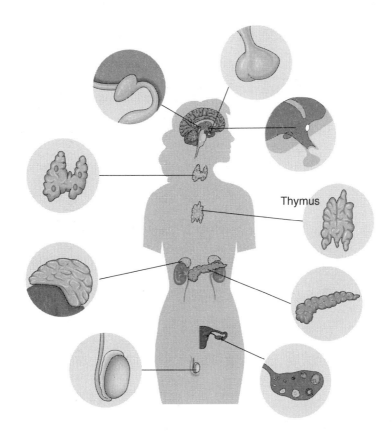

Thymus

    a. How does negative feedback affect hormone production?

    _____

    _____

    b. Name the hormone(s) responsible for each of these functions.

    _____ Increases metabolic rate

    _____ Prolongs the sympathetic nervous response to stress

    _____ Increases blood glucose (two)

    _____ Stimulates growth

    _____ Regulates electrolyte and fluid homeostasis

    _____ Stimulates milk secretion with pregnancy

    _____ Alters blood calcium concentration (two)

    _____ Stimulates uterine contractions

c. What factors make assessment of the endocrine system difficult?

_____

_____

2. List signs/symptoms for the following disorders and briefly describe their treatment.

	Signs/Symptoms	*Treatment*
Acromegaly		
Diabetes insipidus		
Hyperthyroidism		
Hypothyroidism		
Addison's disease		

3. List several risk factors for type 2 diabetes.

(1) _____

(2) _____

(3) _____

(4) _____

(5) _____

(6) _____

a. Which of these clients would be given a diagnosis of diabetes mellitus?
Client A: Has a random blood sugar of 150, asymptomatic
Client B: Has a fasting blood sugar of 130
Client C: Two hours after GTT, has a blood sugar of 180

b. Compare the etiology and management of type 1 and type 2 diabetes.

	Type 1	*Type 2*
Etiology		
Management		

c. Your 21-year-old client was recently diagnosed with type 1 diabetes. He was an avid bicyclist before his diagnosis and is eager to return to competitive racing next season. What guidelines should he follow?

_____

_____

d. Your client with type 1 diabetes describes feeling ill with a mild case of flu. How should she manage her diabetes during the illness?

_____

_____

e. Compare signs and symptoms for the following acute complications of diabetes.

Hypoglycemia: _____

_____

Diabetic ketoacidosis (DKA): _____

_____

HHNK _____

_____

f. List several long-term complications of diabetes.

(1) _____   (5) _____

(2) _____   (6) _____

(3) _____   (7) _____

(4) _____   (8) _____

g. What special concerns are associated with older adults who are diabetic?

_____

_____

4. Nikki, a 25-year-old special education teacher with one toddler at home, has developed a problem with acne and hirsutism, and an irregular menstrual cycle. Although Nikki readily admits that feeling tired by the end of the school day is typical for her, lately the weariness seems to start earlier and earlier. Last week she even felt a little weak. Her family has mentioned to her that she seems to be unusually moody. Physically, her face is looking more full, but she has not gained any weight to account for it. An examination indicates Nikki may have Cushing's syndrome.

a. What is the normal function of the adrenal gland?

_____

_____

b. Describe the causes of adrenal hyperfunction.

_____

_____

c. What other physical and psychological signs and symptoms could Nikki experience?

_____

_____

_____

_____

d. Following a discovery of a growth on her left adrenal gland, Nikki was scheduled for an adrenalectomy. What nursing observations will be needed following her surgery?

_____

_____

e. If steroid therapy is prescribed, what client teaching would you include?

_____

_____

_____

_____

Self-Assessment Questions

Circle the letter that corresponds to the best answer for each question.

1. While reviewing the nursing care for the client who had a removal of the parathyroid glands, the student nurse recalls that a major function of this gland is to
   a. regulate the concentration of blood calcium.
   b. assist the thyroid in regulation of metabolism.
   c. produce a sympathetic nervous response to stress.
   d. stimulate production of stress hormones by the adrenals.

2. The nurse is reviewing care with the nursing student for a client with SIADH. The nurse explains that an important part of the therapeutic management of this syndrome is
   a. frequent oral care.
   b. water restriction and diuretics.
   c. sodium restriction and IV fluids.
   d. monitoring for signs of infection.

3. A client who was diagnosed previously with type 2 diabetes is now using insulin. Two hours before dinner, the client exhibits diaphoresis and anxiety, with a blood glucose of 66. This client would benefit most by
   a. eating two packets of sugar quickly.
   b. asking the physician to adjust the insulin dosage.
   c. having a small glass of juice and an ounce of cheese.
   d. trying to remain calm because anxiety produces the other symptoms.

4. The nurse is performing an assessment on a client with a diagnosis of Addison's disease. Which of the following signs or symptoms would the nurse anticipate?
   a. Bronze coloring and fatigue
   b. Muscle tremors and insomnia
   c. Positive Trousseau's and Chvostek's signs
   d. Moon face and purple striae on the abdomen

5. A nurse is caring for a client following a thyroidectomy. To monitor for the most serious complication of this surgery, the nurse will
   a. monitor the serum calcium levels.
   b. perform voice checks every 2 to 4 hours.
   c. check for respiratory distress and bleeding.
   d. notify the physician of a sore throat or hoarseness.

Nursing Care of the Client: Gastrointestinal System

Chapter

28

Key Terms

Match the following terms with their correct definitions.

___ 1. Adhesion

___ 2. Appendicitis

___ 3. Ascites

___ 4. Calculus

___ 5. Cholecystitis

___ 6. Cholelithiasis

___ 7. Chyme

___ 8. Cirrhosis

___ 9. Colostomy

___10. Constipation

___11. Digestion

___12. Diverticula

___13. Diverticulitis

___14. Diverticulosis

___15. Effluent

___16. Gastric Ulcer

___17. Gastritis

___18. Glycogenesis

___19. Glycogenolysis

a. Saclike protrusion of the intestinal wall that results when the mucosa herniates through the bowel wall.

b. Inflammation of the stomach mucosa.

c. Yellow discoloration of the skin, sclera, mucous membranes, and body fluids that occurs when the liver is unable to fully remove bilirubin from the blood.

d. Stool containing partially broken down blood; usually black, sticky, and tarlike.

e. Erosion formed in the esophagus, stomach, or duodenum resulting from acid/pepsin imbalance.

f. Inflammation of the peritoneum, the membranous covering of the abdomen.

g. Distal end of the gastrointestinal or urinary system brought to the outside of the body and sutured into place.

h. Scar tissue from previous surgeries or disease processes.

i. Abnormal accumulation of fluid in the peritoneal cavity.

j. Process of breaking down complex foods into simple nutrients the body can absorb and convert into energy.

k. Inflammation of one or more diverticula.

l. Liquid output from an ileostomy.

m. Test for microscopic blood done on stool.

n. Inflammation of the oral mucosa.

o. Saclike pouches of the colon.

p. Conversion of glycogen into glucose.

q. Erosion in the stomach.

r. Concentration of mineral salts in the body leading to the formation of stone.

s. Presence of gallstones or calculi in the gallbladder.

___20. Haustra

t. Opening created in the small intestine at the ileum.

___21. Hematemesis

u. Vomiting of blood.

___22. Hemorrhoid

v. Abnormal growth of tissue.

___23. Hepatitis

w. Inflammation of the vermiform appendix.

___24. Ileostomy

x. Inflammation of the gallbladder.

___25. Intussusception

y. Condition characterized by hard, infrequent stools that are difficult or painful to pass.

___26. Jaundice

z. Condition in which multiple diverticula are present in the colon.

___27. Ligation

aa. Conversion of glucose into glycogen.

___28. Melena

bb. Application of a band or tie around a structure.

___29. Occult Blood Test (Guaiac)

cc. Coordinated, rhythmic, serial contraction of the smooth muscles of the gastrointestinal tract.

___30. Pancreatitis

dd. Fatty stool.

___31. Peptic Ulcer

ee. Mixture of partially digested food and digestive enzymes.

___32. Peristalsis

ff. Swollen vascular tissue in the rectal area.

___33. Peritonitis

gg. Acute or chronic inflammation of the pancreas.

___34. Polyp

hh. After eating.

___35. Postprandial

ii. Twisting of a bowel on itself.

___36. Steatorrhea

jj. Chronic or acute inflammation of the liver.

___37. Stoma

kk. Surgically created opening from the colon through the abdominal wall.

___38. Stomatitis

ll. Chronic degenerative changes in the liver cells and thickening of surrounding tissue.

___39. Volvulus

mm. Telescoping of one part of the intestine into another.

Abbreviation Review

Write the definition of the following abbreviations and acronyms.

1. ALT _____

2. AST _____

3. CBD _____

4. CEA _____

5. CHF _____

6. EGD _____

7. ET _____

8. GERD _____

9. GGT _____

10. H & H _____

11. HAV _____

12. HBIG _____

13. HCl _____

14. HCV _____

15. HDV _____

16. IBD _____

17. LDH _____

18. LES _____

19. NG _____

20. NPO _____

21. NSAID _____

22. OTC _____

23. PT _____

24. PTT _____

25. RLQ _____

26. TIPS _____

27. UC _____

28. UGI _____

29. VS _____

Exercises and Activities

1. Label this diagram of the digestive system.

> Appendix
>
> Ascending colon
>
> Descending colon
>
> Duodenum
>
> Esophagus
>
> Gallbladder
>
> Ileum
>
> Jejunum
>
> Liver
>
> Pancreas
>
> Rectum
>
> Salivary glands
>
> Sigmoid
>
> Stomach
>
> Transverse colon

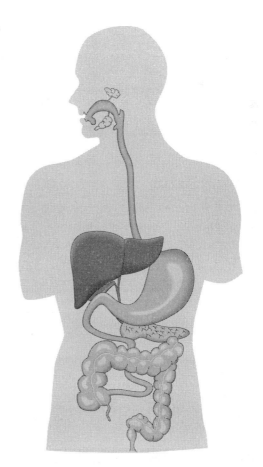

a. Identify two or more functions for each of the following:

Mouth

(1) _____

(2) _____

Gallbladder

(1) _____

(2) _____

Small intestine

(1) _____

(2) _____

Large intestine

(1) _____

(2) _____

Stomach

(1) _____

(2) _____

(3) _____

Pancreas

(1) _____

(2) _____

(3) _____

Liver

(1) _____

(2) _____

(3) _____

(4) _____

(5) _____

b. What changes with aging in the older adult make good nutrition more difficult?

_____

_____

_____

_____

2. If your client has gastrointestinal symptoms, what types of questions will you ask the client?

_____

_____

_____

a. What information will be obtained from the physical examination?

_____

_____

3. Compare symptoms and medical-surgical management for the following GI disorders.

Disorder	Signs/Symptoms	Management/Interventions
Gastric ulcer		
Hepatitis		
Cirrhosis		
Oral cancer		

a. What are predisposing factors for developing peritonitis? What objective findings might be present?

_____

_____

b. Briefly describe treatment/interventions for the client with peritonitis.

_____

_____

4. What strategies might help a client manage the following GI symptoms?

Constipation: _____

_____

Anorexia: _____

_____

a. How can health care workers protect themselves from acquiring hepatitis?

_____

_____

5. Mr. Bernhardt is a 38-year-old security officer with a small home security company. He is being seen for chronic gastrointestinal symptoms. Over the past 3 years, he has been experiencing cramping and abdominal pain and a weight loss of several pounds. He sometimes has several loose stools a day and is now having occasional bloody diarrhea. Other than his own food allergies, he is not aware of any particular family history of gastrointestinal disease. After previously being diagnosed with ulcerative colitis, he was given medication that has been only partially helpful. Now, his increasing bouts of pain and diarrhea are making it very difficult for him to work.

a. How does ulcerative colitis differ from Crohn's disease?

_____

_____

b. What dietary/lifestyle changes might help a client with ulcerative colitis?

_____

_____

c. What are the goals for management of this disease?

_____

_____

d. Because medication and dietary management have been unsuccessful in controlling Mr. Bernhardt's symptoms, what surgical intervention might be indicated?

_____

_____

e. If untreated, what complications is he at risk for? What complications is a client with Crohn's disease at risk of developing?

_____

_____

f. How does inflammatory bowel disease impact an individual's life?

_____

_____

Self-Assessment Questions

Circle the letter that corresponds to the best answer for each question.

1. The nurse's assessment findings for the client with gastrointestinal bleeding may include hematemesis and a black, sticky, tarlike stool called
   a. guaiac.
   b. melena.
   c. steatorrhea.
   d. meconium.

2. The process of converting glycogen to glucose in response to low blood sugar is a function of the
   a. liver.
   b. pancreas.
   c. duodenum.
   d. gallbladder.

3. Your client has been diagnosed with infectious hepatitis. As the nurse caring for this client, you understand that to decrease your chance of acquiring this disease, you need to
   a. avoid needle sticks.
   b. use enteric precautions.
   c. use a gown and special respiratory mask.
   d. complete the hepatitis B immunization series.

4. A client is admitted with a gastrointestinal disorder. She complains of pain in the upper right quadrant that radiates to the right scapular area 2 hours after eating. She now has nausea and indigestion. The nurse recalls that these are symptoms of
   a. gastritis.
   b. appendicitis.
   c. cholecystitis.
   d. irritable bowel syndrome.

5. A nurse is performing an assessment on a client with a gastric ulcer in the duodenum. The nurse may anticipate symptoms that include pain 2 to 4 hours after eating, pain during the night, and
   a. fatigue.
   b. diarrhea.
   c. weight loss.
   d. weight gain.

6. For the client being treated for ulcers, the physician orders antacids, prostaglandins, and
   a. Indocin.
   b. NSAIDs.
   c. H₂ blockers.
   d. milk products.

Nursing Care of the Client: Urinary System

Key Terms

Match the following terms with their correct definitions.

___ 1. Anasarca

___ 2. Azotemia

___ 3. Cachectic

___ 4. Calculus

___ 5. Cystitis

___ 6. Dialysate

___ 7. Dialysis

___ 8. Dysuria

___ 9. Erythropoiesis

___ 10. Fulguration

___ 11. Ideal Conduit

___ 12. Intravesical

___ 13. Litholapaxy

___ 14. Lithotripsy

___ 15. Micturition

___ 16. Nephrotoxic

___ 17. Nocturnal Enuresis

___ 18. Overflow Incontinence

a. Inability to suppress the sudden urge or need to urinate.

b. Pus in the urine.

c. Within the urinary bladder.

d. Calculus or stone formed in the urinary tract.

e. Difficult or painful urination.

f. Generalized edema.

g. Method of crushing a calculus any place in the urinary system with ultrasonic waves.

h. Production of red blood cells and their release by the red bone marrow.

i. Nitrogenous wastes present in the blood.

j. Mechanical means of removing nitrogenous waste from the blood by imitating the function of the nephrons; involves filtration and diffusion of wastes, drugs, and excess electrolytes and/or osmosis of water across a semipermeable membrane into a dialysate solution.

k. Implantation of the ureters into a piece of ileum, which is attached to the abdominal wall as a stoma so urine can be removed from the body.

l. Behind the peritoneum outside the peritoneal cavity.

m. Severe pain in the kidney that radiates to the groin.

n. Concentration of mineral salts, known as stones.

o. Process of expelling the urine from the urinary bladder; also called urination or voiding.

p. Crushing of a bladder stone and immediate washing out of the fragments through a catheter.

q. Bacterial infection of the renal pelvis, tubules, and interstitial tissue of one or both kidneys.

r. Being in a state of malnutrition and wasting.

___19. Pyelonephritis

___20. Pyuria

___21. Renal Colic

___22. Residual Urine

___23. Retroperitoneal

___24. Stress Incontinence

___25. Urge Incontinence

___26. Urinary Incontinence

___27. Urinary Retention

___28. Urolithiasis

s. Incontinence that occurs during sleep.

t. Solution used in dialysis, designed to approximate the normal electrolyte structure of plasma and extracellular fluid.

u. Leakage of urine when a person does anything that strains the abdomen, such as coughing, laughing, jogging, dancing, sneezing, lifting, making a quick movement, or even walking.

v. Leaking of urine when the bladder becomes very full and distended.

w. Urine remaining in the bladder after the individual has urinated.

x. Involuntary loss of urine from the bladder.

y. Procedure to destroy tissue with long high-frequency electric sparks.

z. Inability to void when there is an urge to void.

aa. Inflammation of the urinary bladder.

bb. Quality of a substance that causes kidney tissue damage.

Abbreviation Review

Write the definition of the following abbreviations and acronyms.

1. ACKD _____
2. ACS _____
3. AML _____
4. ARF _____
5. ATN _____
6. A-V _____
7. BPH _____
8. C&S _____
9. CAPD _____
10. EABV _____
11. ESR _____
12. ESRD _____
13. ESWL _____
14. GFR _____
15. NIDDK _____
16. NSAID _____
17. PKD _____
18. ROM _____
19. TIU _____

Exercises and Activities

1. What are the four functions of the kidneys?

   (1) _____

   (2) _____

   (3) _____

   (4) _____

   a. Draw the kidneys, ureters, and bladder in the correct location on the diagram.

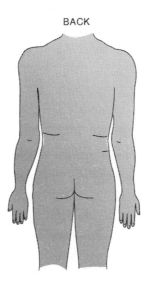

BACK

   b. List six warning signs for kidney disease.

   (1) _____

   (2) _____

   (3) _____

   (4) _____

   (5) _____

   (6) _____

   c. What changes in older adults make them more prone to having problems with urination, infection, and kidney failure?

   _____

   _____

   _____

   _____

2. Which clients need a more thorough assessment of the urinary system?

_____

_____

_____

   a. Identify several subjective and objective assessment findings for clients with kidney disorders.

     _____

     _____

     _____

   b. What terms would be used to document these findings?

     Pus in the urine_____

     Painful urination_____

     Blood in the urine_____

   c. A client on your rehabilitation unit tells you one morning, "It hurts when I urinate." Write five questions that you might ask to get more information.

     (1) _____

     (2) _____

     (3) _____

     (4) _____

     (5) _____

3. List medical, surgical, or lifestyle interventions for the following symptoms.

	Interventions
Stress incontinence	
Nocturnal enuresis	
Urge incontinence	

   a. Which clients are predisposed for developing renal calculi? What signs and symptoms might they experience?

     _____

     _____

   b. Briefly describe two forms of medical-surgical treatment for calculi.

     _____

     _____

     _____

     _____

4. Your client, who is 29 years old, has developed chronic renal failure because of an inherited polycystic kidney disease. As she waits for a transplant, what information will she need about her diet and activity?

_____

_____

_____

   a. How would you explain the differences between peritoneal dialysis and hemodialysis?

     _____

     _____

     _____

     _____

   b. What special precautions are needed for a client who uses hemodialysis?

     _____

     _____

     _____

     _____

     _____

5. Keith Wilson, a 22-year-old junior programmer at a local computer firm, missed a few days of work 2 weeks ago with a bad sore throat and a fever. He thought he had a mild case of flu because several co-workers had been out sick with it recently. Keith is usually a cheerful, easy-going guy, but now he feels miserable with a headache, no appetite, and malaise, and he thinks his urine looks a little odd. Keith says he should be over the flu by now, "so what's wrong with me?"

   a. Keith is suspected of having acute glomerulonephritis, a disorder frequently caused by which one of the following?

     Klebsiella   *Haemophilus influenzae*

     Escherichia coli   *Pseudomonas aeruginosa*

     Staphylococcus aureus   *group A β-hemolytic streptococcus*

   b. Is this an upper UTI or a lower UTI? _____

   c. What other signs and symptoms might Keith have?

     _____

     _____

   d. What laboratory results would you anticipate with acute glomerulonephritis?

     _____

     _____

e. Keith says he doesn't understand how a throat infection could give him a kidney problem. How will you explain this to him?

_____

_____

f. Keith wants to know what the treatment is for his disorder. Discuss medical interventions, including medication, diet, and activity.

_____

_____

_____

_____

_____

g. If Keith's kidney disorder becomes chronic, what long-term symptoms and signs would he experience? What would be the treatment?

_____

_____

_____

_____

_____

_____

Self-Assessment Questions

Circle the letter that corresponds to the best answer for each question.

1. A nursing student is reviewing the care of a client who is experiencing renal failure. The student recalls that functions of the kidney include helping with acid-base balance, secreting renin to raise blood pressure, and producing a hormone responsible for
   a. sodium excretion.
   b. serum calcium levels.
   c. adrenal gland stimulation.
   d. red blood cell production.

2. During morning report to the student, the nurse states that a client with acute renal failure now has oliguria. The student understands that this indicates the client is
   a. having pain with urination.
   b. voiding less than 400 mL per day.
   c. voiding more than 1,000 mL per day.
   d. voiding fewer than four times in 24 hours.

3. Fluid restriction will be an appropriate intervention for the client with a diagnosis of
   a. ESRD.
   b. urolithiasis.
   c. pyelonephritis.
   d. urge incontinence.

4. A nurse is providing discharge instructions to a client who has received treatment for urinary calcium calculi. Which of the following statements by the client indicates a need for additional teaching?
   a. "I need to keep track of my intake and output."
   b. "I should drink plenty of water and other fluids every day."
   c. "Too much activity and exercise can make more stones form."
   d. "Milk and other dairy products may cause me to have more stones."

5. The nursing student is assigned to care for a client with kidney failure who receives hemodialysis using an arteriovenous graft. Which of the following will the instructor emphasize to the student?
   a. Weigh the client before and after each dialysis treatment.
   b. Medications should be administered shortly before dialysis.
   c. Absence of a thrill or bruit over the graft site is a normal finding.
   d. Take the blood pressure and pulse on the arm with the graft to assess for circulation.

Nursing Care of the Client: Female Reproductive System

Key Terms

Match the following terms with their correct definitions.

___ 1. Abortion

___ 2. Amenorrhea

___ 3. Contraception

___ 4. Cystocele

___ 5. Dysmenorrhea

___ 6. Dyspareunia

___ 7. Endometriosis

___ 8. Infertility

___ 9. Menopause

___10. Menorrhagia

___11. Metrorrhagia

___12. Oligomenorrhea

___13. Polymenorrhea

___14. Prolapsed Uterus

___15. Rectocele

___16. Tenesmus

___17. Urethrocele

a. Painful intercourse.

b. Inability or diminished ability to produce offspring.

c. Termination of pregnancy before the age of fetal viability, usually 24 weeks.

d. Menstrual periods that are abnormally frequent, generally less than every 21 days.

e. Spasmodic contradiction of the anal or bladder sphincter, causing pain and a persistent urge to empty the bowel or bladder.

f. Downward displacement of the bladder into the anterior vaginal wall.

g. Absence of menstruation.

h. Cessation of menstruation.

i. Downward displacement of the urethra into the vagina.

j. Growth of endometrial tissue on structures outside of the uterus, within the pelvic cavity.

k. Vaginal bleeding between menstrual periods.

l. Measure taken to prevent pregnancy.

m. Downward displacement of the uterus into the vagina.

n. Painful menstruation.

o. Excessively heavy menstrual flow.

p. Decreased menstrual flow.

q. Anterior displacement of the rectum into the posterior vaginal wall.

Abbreviation Review

Write the definition of the following abbreviations and acronyms.

1. AP _____
2. BSE _____
3. CIS _____
4. CPAP _____
5. D&C _____
6. DES _____
7. ERT _____
8. FBD _____
9. FSH _____
10. GIFT _____
11. IUD _____
12. IVP _____
13. KUB _____
14. LH _____
15. PID _____
16. PMS _____
17. STD _____
18. TSS _____
19. ZIFT _____

Exercises and Activities

1. Label the following diagrams of the female reproductive system.

    Adipose tissue

    Areola

    Cooper's ligament

    Glandular tissue

    Lactiferous duct

    Lobes

    Montgomery tubercles

    Nipple

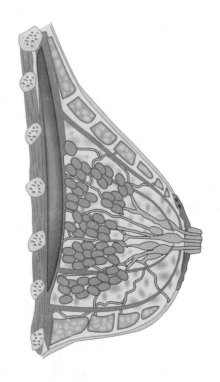

Cervix

Clitoris

Fallopian tube

Fimbriae

Ovary

Symphysis pubis

Urethra

Urinary bladder

Uterus

Vagina

2. Describe the life cycle of an ovum from the time it ripens until implantation occurs (with pregnancy) and the influence of hormones.

_____

_____

_____

_____

   a. What changes take place if implantation does not occur?

     _____

     _____

3. Compare the following breast lesions: cyst, fibroadenoma, and carcinoma.

	Shape	*Mobility*	*Tenderness*	*Erythema*	*Retraction*
Cyst					
Fibroadenoma					
Carcinoma					

a. Marsha, a 31-year-old woman in your clinic, tells you that a close friend of hers was just diagnosed with breast cancer. Although Marsha occasionally has breast and pelvic exams done at the clinic, she has never really wanted to learn breast self-examination until now. How will you instruct her to perform BSE? What will you tell her about the frequency and timing for BSE?

_____

_____

_____

_____

_____

_____

b. List nine risk factors for breast cancer.

(1) _____   (6) _____

(2) _____   (7) _____

(3) _____   (8) _____

(4) _____   (9) _____

(5) _____

4. Compare the signs/symptoms and the primary treatment for the following disorders.

	Signs/Symptoms	*Treatment*
Pelvic inflammatory disease (PID)		
Endometriosis		
Ovarian cancer		
Prolapsed uterus		

a. List several risk factors for cervical cancer.

(1) _____

(2) _____

(3) _____

(4) _____

b. How does toxic shock syndrome (TSS) develop?

_____

_____

_____

5. A female client has determined that she would like to use the "rhythm method" of contraception. What information will she need? What might be the risks/side effects and advantages of this method?

_____

_____

_____

_____

a. Which methods of contraception require the client to be seen by a health care provider?

_____

_____

_____

b. List methods of contraception that may offer some protection against STDs.

_____

_____

_____

6. Ms. Collins, a 48-year-old office administrator, has an appointment today at your clinic. Over the past few months, she has noticed that her menstrual cycle is changing. She has also noticed feeling some nervousness and mood swings. At first she attributed her symptoms to a recent promotion and increased responsibility. Now Ms. Collins is also having occasional "hot flashes" that wake her up at night. She is here for a Pap smear and wants to talk about hormone replacement therapy.

a. What physical changes occur with menopause?

_____

_____

_____

_____

b. What subjective and objective data will be obtained during the assessment?

_____

_____

_____

_____

c. List advantages and disadvantages of hormone replacement therapy.

_____

_____

_____

_____

_____

d. What steps can Ms. Collins take to maintain or improve her health?

_____

_____

_____

e. Ms. Collins states, "Well, at least I won't be needing any more pelvic exams now." What will you tell your client? How does her risk for breast cancer change?

_____

_____

_____

Self-Assessment Questions

Circle the letter that corresponds to the best answer for each question.

1. A female client is recently diagnosed with infertility related to a hormone imbalance. To treat infertility for this client, the physician orders
   a. Clomid.
   b. Norplant.
   c. Progesterone.
   d. Depo-Provera.

2. A client has just had a modified mastectomy for breast cancer. To help the client adjust to the loss of her breast, the nurse will
   a. expect the client to assume self-care after the surgery.
   b. assess breath sounds, vital signs, and provide O_2 as needed.
   c. encourage the client to look at the surgical site when she is ready.
   d. assist the client to do active ROM exercises to strengthen the affected side.

3. The nurse is assessing a client with a diagnosis of fibroid tumors. The nurse anticipates that this client may report pelvic pressure, abdominal enlargement, bleeding between menstrual periods, and an excessively heavy menstrual flow called
   a. hematuria.
   b. menorrhagia.
   c. hematemesis.
   d. dysmenorrhea.

4. Your client, who is 36 years old and married, asks for information about birth control methods. She definitely wants to avoid another pregnancy but isn't ready for sterilization. You are aware from her health history that she smokes. Which of the following options would be most appropriate?

   a. Depo-Provera
   b. Rhythm method
   c. Oral contraceptives
   d. Foam or gel spermicides

5. After her routine gynecological exam, your client, who is 47 years old, asks you about changes that she will experience with menopause. Which of the following would not be included in your teaching?

   a. Menstruation will cease.
   b. Stress incontinence may occur.
   c. Risk for osteoporosis will increase.
   d. Skin turgor and elasticity will increase.

Nursing Care of the Client: Male Reproductive System

Key Terms

Match the following terms with their correct definitions.

___ 1. Hematuria

___ 2. Hesitancy

___ 3. Impotence

___ 4. Nocturia

___ 5. Orchiectomy

___ 6. Post Void Residual

___ 7. Priapism

___ 8. Spermatogenesis

___ 9. Urethrostomy

___10. Vasectomy

a. Production of sperm.

b. Awakening at night to void.

c. Surgical resection of the vas deferens.

d. Difficulty initiating the urinary stream.

e. Prolonged erection that does not occur in response to sexual stimulation.

f. Formation of a permanent fistula opening into the urethra.

g. Blood in the urine.

h. Inability of an adult male to have an erection firm enough, or to maintain it long enough, to complete sexual intercourse.

i. Urine that remains in the bladder after urination.

j. Removal of a testis.

Abbreviation Review

Write the definition of the following abbreviations and acronyms.

1. AAP _____

2. B&O _____

3. BPH _____

4. BSE _____

5. DES _____

6. DICC _____

7. FSH _____

8. LH _____

9. PSA _____

10. STD _____

11. TSE _____

12. TULIP _____

13. TURP _____

14. UTI _____

15. VCD _____

Exercises and Activities

1. Label the following diagram of the male reproductive system.

Cowper's glands

Ejaculatory duct

Epididymis

Glans penis

Prepuce (foreskin)

Prostate gland

Scrotum

Seminal vesicle

Testis

Urethra

Vas deferens

a. How are sperm produced and released? What is the role of hormones?

_____

_____

_____

2. What are the risk factors and symptoms for testicular cancer?

_____

_____

_____

a. How would you describe the testicular self-exam (TSE) to your male client?

_____

_____

_____

b. Compare the signs and symptoms and the primary treatment for the following disorders.

	Signs/Symptoms	*Treatment*
Orchitis		
Prostate Cancer		
BPH		

c. List several possible causes of impotence for the male client.

_____

_____

_____

d. Describe one method of treatment for impotence.

_____

_____

_____

3. A male client has determined that he will use the condom for contraception. What information will he need to use it appropriately? What are the advantages of this method?

_____

_____

_____

4. Mr. Thurmond, a 57-year-old African-American, has come in today for a routine physical examination, which he does "every few years or so." During the health history, Mr. Thurmond also mentions that he has been having a little hesitancy and straining when he urinates. More recently, he also noticed a reduction in his urinary stream. Since an older brother was diagnosed a year ago with benign prostatic hypertrophy (BPH) and had similar symptoms, he hasn't been too worried about it. He's really more concerned about his blood pressure right now, and wants to get it checked.

a. Compare the symptoms of BPH and prostate cancer.

_____

_____

_____

b. Mr. Thurmond asks you what tests he needs to check his prostate gland. Identify several tests that might be indicated.

_____

_____

_____

c. At a follow-up visit, Mr. Thurmond is advised he has prostate cancer in an early stage. What other signs or symptoms might be noted in a client with this disease?

_____

_____

_____

d. What are the risk factors for prostate cancer?

(1) _____

(2) _____

(3) _____

(4) _____

e. One of the treatments being considered for Mr. Thurmond is cryosurgical ablation. Briefly describe this procedure for your client.

_____

_____

_____

f. What nursing observations would be needed following surgery for Mr. Thurmond?

_____

_____

_____

Self-Assessment Questions

Circle the letter that corresponds to the best answer for each question.

1. A male client with which of the following conditions would require immediate surgery?
   a. varicocele
   b cryptorchidism
   c. prostatic hypertrophy
   d. torsion of the spermatic cord

2. The nurse is instructing a 20-year-old male client to perform testicular self-exam (TSE) to screen for testicular cancer. The instructions to the client include performing the exam after a bath or shower and noting any
   a. difficulty with urination.
   b. small, hard, painless lumps.
   c. painful, swollen lymph nodes.
   d. worm-like mass in the scrotum.

3. A 45-year-old male client is having a routine physical examination. For this client, the most useful screening method to detect prostate cancer is
   a. a rectal examination performed annually.
   b. a serum prostate specific antigen (PSA) test.
   c. observation of symptoms such as hematuria.
   d. monthly self-exam for painless lumps in the testes.

4. Your male client is using condoms for contraception and protection against STDs. Which of the following actions shows a need for further instruction?
   a. Using latex condoms
   b. Leaving an inch at the tip of the condom
   c. Applying the condom just prior to ejaculation
   d. Unrolling the condom over the penis to apply

5. Counseling for sexual dysfunction is especially important for the client with prostate cancer who is being treated with
   a. hormonal agents.
   b. cryosurgical ablation.
   c. radioactive seed implants.
   d. surgical removal of the gland.

Nursing Care of the Client: Sexually Transmitted Diseases

Chapter

32

Key Terms

Match the following terms with their correct definitions.

___ 1. Antibiotic-Resistant

___ 2. Chancre

___ 3. Chlamydia

___ 4. Cytomegalovirus

___ 5. Exposure

___ 6. Gonorrhea

___ 7. Incidence

___ 8. Incubation Period

___ 9. Syphilis

___10. Trichomoniasis

___11. Venereal Disease

a. Sexually transmitted disease caused by a parasitic protozoan, *Trichomonas vaginalis.*

b. Sexually transmitted disease caused by the gram-negative bacterial organism *Neisseria gonorrhea.*

c. Disease usually acquired as a result of sexual contact; the preferred term currently in use is sexually transmitted disease.

d. Sexually transmitted disease caused by the spherical bacterial organism *Chlamydia trachomatis.*

e. Resistant to a previously effective antimicrobial agent.

f. One of the herpes type viruses; inhabits saliva, urine, blood, semen, and vaginal secretions.

g. Frequency of disease occurrence.

h. Sexually transmitted disease caused by the spirochete *Treponema pallidum.*

i. Clean, painless, syphilitic, primary ulcer appearing 2 to 6 weeks after infection at the site of body contact.

j. Contact with an infected person or agent.

k. Interval between exposure to an infectious disease and the first appearance of symptoms.

Abbreviation Review

Write the definition of the following acronyms.

1. AIDS _____

2. CMV _____

3. ELISA _____

4. HBV _____

5. HIV _____

6. HPV _____

7. HSV _____

8. PID _____

9. RPR _____

10. STD _____

11. VDRL _____

Exercises and Activities

1. Describe the role of the nurse in the identification and treatment of sexually transmitted diseases (STDs).

_____

_____

_____

   a. What information would be gathered in the client interview?

_____

_____

_____

   b. List signs and symptoms frequently noted in the client with a sexually transmitted disease.

_____

_____

_____

   c. How can the nurse help the client feel more comfortable during the interview and physical assessment?

_____

_____

2. What factors have contributed to an increase in the frequency of STDs?

_____

_____

_____

   a. Why is education important in prevention of STDs?

_____

_____

   b. You are asked to help prepare an educational program for high school–age students on prevention of STDs. What topics will you include?

_____

_____

_____

c. What will you advise the students to do if they feel they have been exposed to a sexually transmitted disease?

_____

_____

3. Describe the signs and symptoms and treatment for each of the following STDs.

Disease	Signs/Symptoms	Treatment
Genital herpes		
Gonorrhea		
Genital warts		
Trichomoniasis		

a. Why are STDs more dangerous for female clients?

_____

_____

4. Ryan, a 23-year-old single male client, is being seen at the clinic for a small painless ulcer on the end of his penis. He first noticed it last week and thought it would go away, but when it didn't he decided to get it checked. Ryan admits having sexual relations with three different partners within the past several months. He says he probably should be using condoms, but his current girlfriend is on birth control pills. Ryan denies burning on urination, penile discharge, fever, rash, or other symptoms. Assessment findings include regional lymphadenopathy. Results on VDRL and FTA-ABS tests indicate syphilis.

a. List signs and symptoms for each stage of syphilis.

Primary: _____

_____

Secondary: _____

_____

Latent: _____

_____

Tertiary: _____

_____

b. What stage of syphilis is Ryan probably in? _____

Which stage is most contagious? _____

What medication will be used to treat Ryan? _____

c. Why is syphilis called "the great imitator"?

_____

_____

d. What information does Ryan need about follow-up care, sexual activity, and risk for STDs?

_____

_____

Self-Assessment Questions

Circle the letter that corresponds to the best answer for each question.

1. A female client with genital warts is receiving treatment to have them removed. When instructing the client about this sexually transmitted disease, the nurse emphasizes that the client
   a. will need frequent Pap smears.
   b. must complete the entire antibiotic therapy.
   c. should avoid sexual activity until she is cured.
   d. will probably not have a recurrence because the warts were removed.

2. Between 80% and 100% of adults have developed antibodies to
   a. CMV.
   b. chlamydia.
   c. hepatitis B.
   d. genital herpes.

3. A male client is diagnosed with secondary syphilis. While assessing this client, the nurse is likely to note
   a. seizures and stroke symptoms.
   b. a single chancre, usually near the tip of the penis.
   c. burning on urination and a discharge from the penis.
   d. a skin rash of small brownish sores, including the palms and soles.

4. The nurse is instructing a client about preventing STDs. Which of these statements by the client indicates a need for additional teaching?
   a. "I won't get STDs if I use a latex condom."
   b. "Even if I have an STD, I may not have any symptoms."
   c. "Hepatitis B is the only STD I can be vaccinated against."
   d. "If I have an STD, my partner and I both need treatment."

5. Factors that have led to an increased number of clients with STDs include all but which of the following?
   a. Increased alcohol and drug use
   b. Use of nonbarrier methods of birth control
   c. Greater awareness of how STDs are transmitted
   d. Increased numbers of teens engaging in sexual activity

6. The nurse is providing care for a client with genital herpes. The nurse remembers that this sexually transmitted disease is
   a. contagious even if there are no symptoms present.
   b. curable if diagnosed early and treated with Acyclovir.
   c. contagious only when blisters are present in the perineal area.
   d. caused by HSV type 1, which also causes "fever blisters" on the lips.

Nursing Care of the Client: Mental Illness

Key Terms

Match the following terms with their correct definitions.

___ 1. Abuse

___ 2. Actively Suicidal

___ 3. Affect

___ 4. Anger-Control Assistance

___ 5. Anorexia Nervosa

___ 6. Anxiety

___ 7. Anxiolytic

___ 8. Auditory Hallucination

___ 9. Brief Dynamic Therapy

___10. Bulimia Nervosa

___11. Cognitive Behavior Therapy

___12. Command Hallucination

a. Laboratory test done to determine whether the client's lithium level is within a therapeutic range.

b. Antianxiety medication.

c. Constantly scanning the environment for potentially dangerous situations.

d. Treatment of mental and emotional disorders through psychological rather than physical methods.

e. Psychiatric disorder characterized by periods of binge eating of up to 10,000 calories at one time followed by self-induced vomiting and other forms of purging such as laxative and diuretic abuse.

f. Stressor that forces an individual to respond and/or adapt in some way.

g. Condition wherein an individual has a distorted view of self, is unable to maintain satisfying personal relationships, and is unable to adapt to the environment.

h. Bond or connection between two people that is based on mutual trust.

i. Procedure whereby clients are treated with pulses of electrical energy sufficient to cause brief convulsions or seizures.

j. Rapid, intense speech.

k. Perception by an individual that someone is talking when no one in fact is there.

l. Treatment approach aimed at helping a client identify stimuli that cause the client's anxiety, develop plans to respond to those stimuli in a nonanxious manner, and problem solve when unanticipated anxiety-provoking situations arise.

___13. Confidentiality

m. Incident involving some type of violation to the client.

___14. Crisis

n. Therapy focused on uncovering unconscious memories and processes.

___15. Cycling

o. Reliving of an original trauma as though the individual were currently experiencing it.

___16. Delusion

p. Mild form of mania without significant impairment.

___17. Depression

q. State wherein an individual experiences feelings of extreme sadness, hopelessness, and helplessness.

___18. Domestic Violence

r. Eating disorder characterized by self-imposed starvation by restricting caloric intake and compulsively exercising.

___19. Electroconvulsive Therapy

s. Nondisclosure of the identity of personal information about an individual.

___20. Empathy

t. Perception by an individual that someone is present when no one is.

___21. Euphoric

u. Purposefully taking one's own life.

___22. Flashback

v. Short-term psychotherapy that focuses on resolving core conflicts deriving from personality and living situations.

___23. Genuineness

w. Perception that something is present when it is not.

___24. Hallucination

x. Extremely elevated mood with accompanying agitated behavior.

___25. Hypersomnia

y. Acquired resistance to the effects of a drug.

___26. Hypervigilant

z. Descriptor of an individual who threatens to or actually harms someone.

___27. Hypomania

aa. State wherein a person feels a strong sense of dread, frequently accompanied by physical symptoms of increased heart and respiratory rates and elevated blood pressure in the absence of a specific source or reason for the emotions or responses.

___28. Insomnia

bb. Ability to perceive and relate to another's personal experience.

___29. Lethargy

cc. Aggression and violence involving family members.

___30. Libido

dd. Descriptor of an individual intent upon hurting or killing self and who is in imminent danger of doing so.

___31. Mania

ee. Acceptance of an individual as is and in a nonjudgmental manner.

___32. Mental Disorder

ff. Difficulty in falling asleep initially or returning to sleep once awakened.

___33. Mental Illness

gg. Perception an individual has of a voice or voices telling the individual to do something, usually to themselves and/or someone else.

___34. Mood

hh. Sexual energy.

___35. Neglect

ii. Overreaction to minor sounds or noises.

___36. Paradoxical Reaction

jj. Confinement of a client to a single room.

___37. Physically Aggressive

kk. Clinically significant behavior or psychological syndrome or pattern that occurs in an individual and is associated with present distress or disability or with a significantly increased risk of suffering, death, pain, disability, or an important loss of freedom (APA, 1994).

___38. Pressured Speech

ll. Alteration in mood between depression and mania.

___39. Psychoanalysis

mm. Outward manifestation of the way an individual is feeling.

___40. Psychosis

nn. Poisonous.

___41. Psychotherapy

oo. Subjective report of the way an individual is feeling.

___42. Rapport

pp. Excessive sleep.

___43. Respect

qq. Opposite effect of that which would normally be expected.

___44. Seclusion

rr. Nursing intervention aimed at facilitating the expression of anger in an adaptive and nonviolent manner.

___45. Serum Lithium Level

ss. False belief that misrepresents reality.

___46. Startle Response

tt. State wherein an individual has lost the ability to recognize reality.

___47. Suicidal Ideation

uu. Characterized by elation out of context to the situation.

___48. Suicide

vv. Thought of hurting or killing oneself.

___49. Tolerance

ww. Ability to rely on an individual's character and ability.

___50. Toxic

xx. Sincerity.

___51. Trust

yy. Decreased energy level.

___52. Verbally Aggressive

zz. Descriptor of an individual who says things in a loud and/or intimidating manner.

___53. Visual Hallucination

aaa. Nonsensical combination of words that is meaningless to others.

___54. Word Salad

bbb. Situation in which a basic need of the client is not being provided.

Abbreviation Review

Write the definition of the following abbreviations and acronyms.

1. ADHD _____

2. APA _____

3. APS _____

4. bid _____

5. CPS _____

6. DSM-IV _____

7. ECT _____

8. EPS _____

9. GAD _____

10. ICU _____

11. MAOI _____

12. mEq/L _____

13. NMS _____

14. OCD _____

15. OTC _____

16. PCP _____

17. PTSD _____

18. SSRI _____

19. TD _____

Exercises and Activities

1. Think of someone you know who you consider to be mentally healthy. Describe the characteristics of that person that you feel demonstrate mental health.

   _____

   _____

   _____

   _____

   a. What is the role of the nurse in the mental health field?

      _____

      _____

      _____

      _____

   b. How would you explain "the therapeutic use of self" to another student?

      _____

      _____

      _____

      _____

c. List the essential components of a therapeutic relationship.

(1) _____   (4) _____

(2) _____   (5) _____

(3) _____

d. How can the nurse develop a trusting relationship with the client?

_____

_____

_____

_____

2. Compare the symptoms for a client with mild anxiety, moderate anxiety, and severe anxiety.

_____

_____

_____

_____

a. What nursing interventions are important for a client experiencing panic anxiety?

_____

_____

_____

_____

b. Review Table 33 in your text, and list several of the most common side effects of anti-anxiety medications.

(1) _____   (4) _____

(2) _____   (5) _____

(3) _____   (6) _____

c. How does cognitive-behavior therapy work in the treatment of anxiety disorders?

_____

_____

_____

_____

d. Identify methods the nurse can use to help a client achieve stress reduction or relaxation.

_____

_____

_____

_____

3. How would you assess a client for potential for aggression?

_____

_____

_____

_____

a. What techniques can be used with the client who is angry?

_____
_____
_____
_____

b. List behavioral clues that might indicate a client is suicidal.

(1) _____   (5) _____
(2) _____   (6) _____
(3) _____   (7) _____
(4) _____   (8) _____

4. Identify the goals of psychosocial and clinical treatment for the client with schizophrenia.

_____
_____
_____
_____

a. What factors make it difficult to treat clients with schizophrenia?

_____
_____
_____
_____

b. Your client has been prescribed Thorazine, a phenothiazine drug. What information will you include in client teaching about this medication?

_____
_____
_____
_____

c. What assessment findings might alert the health care team to abuse or neglect in a client?

_____
_____
_____
_____

5. Nine months ago, Suzanne and her husband lost their 4-month-old baby boy from sudden infant death syndrome (SIDS). Since then, Suzanne has felt overwhelmed with guilt and grief over the loss. She returned to her secretarial job a month after the death but left again when she couldn't seem to keep her mind on her work. Suzanne no longer enjoys visits with friends or baking, a favorite activity. She has lost several pounds and has trouble making even simple decisions. Suzanne sometimes feels that if she were a stronger person, she could pull herself

out of her sadness and move on. Her husband and friends shared her grief at first but they now think she needs to get on with her life. After all, she still has Carey, their 6-year-old daughter.

a. What signs and symptoms of depression do you see in Suzanne?

_____

_____

_____

_____

_____

b. List other symptoms that may be noted in a client with depression.

_____

_____

_____

_____

c. Describe medical and pharmacological treatments for depression.

_____

_____

_____

_____

_____

d. Suzanne was started in outpatient therapy and will be taking Paxil, a selective serotonin reuptake inhibitor (SSRI) to help with her symptoms. List possible side effects she may experience.

(1) _____   (7) _____

(2) _____   (8) _____

(3) _____   (9) _____

(4) _____   (10) _____

(5) _____   (11) _____

(6) _____   (12) _____

e. Why would a dietary consult be helpful for Suzanne?

_____

_____

_____

f. What information will you include in client teaching about Paxil?

_____

_____

_____

_____

_____

Self-Assessment Questions

Circle the letter that corresponds to the best answer for each question.

1. The nurse is performing an assessment on a client who is taking lithium carbonate for bipolar disorder. The nurse notes that the client has anorexia, headache, tinnitus, and confusion. Which of these findings may indicate lithium toxicity?
   a. Tinnitus
   b. Anorexia
   c. Headache
   d. Confusion

2. One of the first symptoms that may be noted in the client with depression is
   a. a change in sleeping patterns.
   b. a decrease in job performance.
   c. a preoccupation with death or dying.
   d. a sudden change in personal appearance or hygiene.

3. A client diagnosed with ADHD has been prescribed Ritalin, a CNS stimulant. Because of the side effects associated with this medication, the client is monitored for
   a. lethargy.
   b. weight loss.
   c. nosebleeds.
   d. increased urination.

4. A nurse has been assigned to care for a client who is identified as being actively suicidal. The highest priority for the nurse will be to
   a. maintain the safety of the client.
   b. supervise the client's medication.
   c. initiate a therapeutic relationship.
   d. document behaviors that indicate self-harm potential.

5. The nurse is discharging a client who is taking Nardil, a monoamine oxidase inhibitor (MAOI), for depression. The client is advised to avoid decongestants to prevent which serious drug-drug reaction?
   a. Liver toxicity
   b. Agranulocytosis
   c. Atrial fibrillation
   d. Hypertensive crisis

Nursing Care of the Client: Substance Abuse

Key Terms

Match the following terms with their correct definitions.

___ 1. Abuse

___ 2. Addiction

___ 3. Behavioral Tolerance

___ 4. Codependent

___ 5. Confabulation

___ 6. Cross-Tolerance

___ 7. Dependence

___ 8. Detoxification

___ 9. Hallucination

___10. Intoxication

___11. Johnsonian Intervention

___12. Misuse

___13. Opisthotonos

___14. Relapse

a. Reliance on a substance to such a degree that abstinence causes functional impairment, physical withdrawal symptoms, and/or psychological craving for the substance.

b. Decreased sensitivity to other substances in the same category.

c. Use of a legal substance for which it was not intended or exceeding the recommended dosage of a drug.

d. Misuse or excessive or improper use of a substance, the absence of which does not cause withdrawal symptoms.

e. Phenomenon whereby a smaller amount of substance will elicit the desired psychic effects.

f. Symptoms produced when a substance on which an individual has dependence is no longer used by that individual.

g. A drug, legal or illegal, that may cause physical or mental impairment.

h. Compensatory adjustments of behavior made under the influence of a particular substance.

i. A reversible effect on the central nervous system soon after the use of a substance.

j. Description for people who live based on what others think of them.

k. Return to a previous behavior or condition.

l. Elimination of a substance from a person's body.

m. The making up of information to fill in memory gaps.

n. Reliance on a substance to such a degree that abstinence causes functional impairment, physical withdrawal symptoms, and/or psychological craving for the substance.

___15. Reverse Tolerance

o. A complete arching of the body with only the head and feet on the bed.

___16. Substance

p. A confrontational approach to a client with a substance problem that lessens the chance of denial and encourages treatment before the client "hits bottom."

___17. Synthesiasis

q. Hearing colors and seeing sounds.

___18. Teratogenic

r. Decreased sensitivity to subsequent doses of the same substance; an increased dose of the substance is needed to produce the same desired effect.

___19. Tolerance

s. Causing abnormal development of the embryo.

___20. Withdrawal

t. Perceiving things that are not present in reality.

Abbreviation Review

Write the definition of the following abbreviations and acronyms.

1. AA _____

2. ADHD _____

3. AWS _____

4. DEA _____

5. DET _____

6. DETOX _____

7. DMT _____

8. DOM _____

9. DSM-IV _____

10. FAE _____

11. FAS _____

12. LSD _____

13. MADD _____

14. MAOI _____

15. MDMA _____

16. NA _____

17. NIDA _____

18. PCP _____

19. ROM _____

20. SADD _____

21. SIDS _____

Exercises and Activities

1. Describe the factors that might predispose an individual to substance abuse.

   Individual factors: _____

   _____

   Family patterns: _____

   _____

   Lifestyle: _____

   _____

   Environmental factors: _____

   _____

   Developmental factors: _____

   _____

   a. What interpersonal skills can protect an individual from substance abuse?

      _____

      _____

      _____

   b. How would you differentiate abuse from addiction?

      _____

      _____

      _____

2. Identify the legislation that took place during each of the following years and describe its effect on substance abuse in the United States.

   1906: _____

   _____

   1914: _____

   _____

   1919: _____

   _____

   1937: _____

   _____

   1970: _____

   _____

a. List diagnostic testing that can be performed to detect drug and alcohol use.

_____

_____

_____

_____

b. What objective data might be noted on assessment of the client with substance abuse?

_____

_____

_____

_____

_____

3. How would you characterize an individual who is codependent? What is the goal of treatment?

_____

_____

_____

_____

a. Identify problems associated with substance misuse in the elderly.

(1) _____

(2) _____

(3) _____

(4) _____

b. What action would you take if you realized a co-worker was impaired?

_____

_____

_____

_____

c. Identify the goals of the peer assistance program.

(1) _____

(2) _____

(3) _____

(4) _____

4. Deana considers herself a typical college sophomore who just enjoys a good party. She didn't really do much drinking until she went away to school. College seemed like the perfect place to meet new people, study hard during the week, and party on the weekends. It wasn't like she had to drive anywhere; there was always a party with alcohol nearby. Last year, Deana drank only on Friday or Saturday. Now she starts in the middle of the week and is binge-drinking most weekends. Her grades are slipping, but not bad enough to get kicked out of school yet. The campus police caught her drunk in public (DIP) a few times, and the college

has advised her to go into counseling. But if she hadn't broken her foot last weekend falling down the stairs drunk, her parents still wouldn't know.

a. What signs and symptoms indicate that Deana has a problem with alcohol?

_____

_____

_____

_____

b. List the physical and psychological effects of alcohol on the individual.

_____

_____

_____

_____

_____

c. At the urging of her parents and college officials, Deana will be starting in an outpatient counseling program. If Deana experiences minor alcohol withdrawal symptoms, what might these include?

(1) _____ (4) _____ (7) _____

(2) _____ (5) _____ (8) _____

(3) _____ (6) _____ (9) _____

d. List drugs that are often used to treat the symptoms of alcohol withdrawal in a client.

(1) _____ (3) _____

(2) _____ (4) _____

e. Identify problems that are associated with long-term alcohol use.

_____

_____

_____

_____

f. What information on life skills and coping mechanisms would you include in client education with Deana?

_____

_____

_____

_____

_____

_____

Self-Assessment Questions

Circle the letter that corresponds to the best answer for each question.

1. The nurse is performing a physical assessment on a client admitted with a diagnosis of alcohol withdrawal syndrome. Which of the following findings would indicate Stage 2 (major) withdrawal?
   a. Confabulation
   b. Hallucinations
   c. Global confusion
   d. Delirium tremens

2. An example of a schedule I drug is
   a. opium.
   b. morphine.
   c. marijuana.
   d. amphetamine.

3. The nurse at the substance abuse treatment center is caring for a client who had been using phencyclidine (PCP). The nurse recalls that treatment for this client will include
   a. monitoring for seizures.
   b. confrontation to control behaviors.
   c. use of disulfiram (Antabuse) as a deterrent.
   d. observing for signs of physical dependence.

4. A sign that a client with substance abuse is achieving social and family recovery occurs when the client
   a. is able to return to work.
   b. develops a relationship with a higher power.
   c. learns to resist social pressure to use the substance.
   d. receives and accepts professional treatment for detoxification.

5. A nurse is reviewing health history information with the wife of a client recently admitted for substance abuse treatment. The nurse suspects that the wife may be codependent based on the observation that she
   a. appears to have low self-esteem.
   b. also shows signs of substance abuse.
   c. requests information on self-help and support groups.
   d. asks multiple questions about the treatment plan for her husband.

Nursing Care of the Older Client

Key Terms

Match the following terms with their correct definitions.

_____ 1. Activities of Daily Living

a. Federal law enacted in 1997 that replaced cost-based reimbursement for care in skilled nursing facilities with a prospective payment system based on client assessment within a resource utilization group system.

_____ 2. Balanced Budget Act

b. Specialty within nursing that addresses and advocates for the special care needs of older adults.

_____ 3. Delirium

c. Basic care activities that include mobility, bathing, hygiene, grooming, dressing, eating, and toileting.

_____ 4. Dementia

d. Federal agency in charge of administering the Medicare program.

_____ 5. Gerontological Nursing

e. Problem of clients taking numerous prescription and over-the-counter medications for the same or various disease processes, with unknown consequences from the resulting combinations of chemical compounds and cumulative side-effects.

_____ 6. Gerontologist

f. Study of the effects of normal aging and age-related diseases on human beings.

_____ 7. Gerontology

g. Cognitive changes or acute confusion of rapid onset (less than 6 months).

_____ 8. Health Care Financing Agency

h. Specialist in gerontology in advanced practice nursing, geriatric psychiatry, medicine, and social services.

_____ 9. Omnibus Budget Reconciliation Act

i. Federal law first enacted in 1989 to provide for rights and clinical guidelines to ensure quality health services for older Americans.

_____10. Polypharmacy

j. Organic brain pathology characterized by losses in intellectual functioning and a slow onset (longer than 6 months).

Abbreviation Review

Write the definition of the following acronyms.

1. AARP _____
2. AD _____
3. ANA _____
4. BBA _____
5. BPH _____
6. CHF _____
7. COPD _____
8. ERT _____
9. HCFA _____
10. NIDDM _____
11. OBRA _____
12. ORIF _____
13. PPS _____
14. PSA _____
15. PVD _____
16. RTI _____
17. RUGS _____
18. SNF _____
19. THA _____
20. TIA _____
21. UTI _____

Exercises and Activities

1. What changes have occurred in U.S. demographics related to the aging population?

_____

_____

_____

   a. How are attitudes toward aging changing in the United States?

_____

_____

_____

   b. Describe the financial challenges that Americans are facing for elder-care services.

_____

_____

_____

c. Your client, who is approaching retirement, tells you that he is not worried about future health care expenses because he will have Medicare and Medicaid coverage once he reaches age 65. What would you tell him?

_____

_____

_____

2. Describe one biological theory and one psychosocial theory of aging.

_____

_____

_____

_____

a. Why is it important to identify individual strengths in the older client?

_____

_____

_____

b. What is polypharmacy and why is it a danger to the health of the older client?

_____

_____

_____

c. List normal physiological changes that occur with aging in each of the following systems.

Urinary _____

_____

Cardiovascular _____

_____

Gastrointestinal _____

_____

Neurological system_____

_____

d. What physical and lifestyle changes cause the older client to be more susceptible to lung infection?

_____

_____

_____

e. What sensory alterations can cause safety issues for the older client?

_____

_____

_____

3. Describe at least four nursing interventions for the client with each of the following disorders.

Peripheral vascular disease   (1) _____

                                           (2) _____

                                           (3) _____

                                           (4) _____

Chronic CHF   (1) _____

                                           (2) _____

                                           (3) _____

                                           (4) _____

Alzheimer's disease   (1) _____

                                           (2) _____

                                           (3) _____

                                           (4) _____

a. Your client is taking digoxin for chronic congestive heart failure. What are your nursing responsibilities for the safe administration of this medication?

_____

_____

_____

4. Mr. Salokis is a 76-year-old former engineer who has been admitted to your long-term care facility. Divorced years ago, he was living in a retirement community until symptoms of advancing Parkinson's disease required him to have more care. Mr. Salokis had done well on his own, always maintaining a sense of humor. He had regular health checkups and screening, walked outside daily until last year, quit smoking many years ago, and had been active in his retirement community. Mr. Salokis did find it difficult, however, to get food and never enjoyed cooking, so he had lost a few pounds recently. His son lives several hours away and is unable to provide the care Mr. Salokis now requires.

a. Identify the strengths that have helped Mr. Salokis maintain his optimal level of functioning.

_____

_____

b. What impairments will you anticipate with this client related to his Parkinson's disease?

_____

_____

_____

c. Mr. Salokis will need assistance with the activities of daily living (ADL). What activities are included in the ADL?

(1) _____   (4) _____   (6) _____

(2) _____   (5) _____   (7) _____

(3) _____

d. How can you help Mr. Salokis with his ADL while still encouraging his independence and self-esteem?

_____

_____

_____

_____

e. Several days after his admission, you notice Mr. Salokis seems a little confused. What can cause problems with mentation?

_____

_____

_____

f. Your nursing assistant says Mr. Salokis has been having urinary incontinence. What problems could this indicate? Identify interventions that might help.

_____

_____

_____

g. How can adequate nutrition be maintained as swallowing becomes more difficult?

_____

_____

_____

h. Mr. Salokis spends most of his time in his room, rarely leaving or socializing with other residents in the facility. Why is social interaction important and what can you do to support him?

_____

_____

_____

Self-Assessment Questions

Circle the letter that corresponds to the best answer for each question.

1. The nurse is reviewing assessment data for an older client recently admitted to a long-term care facility. Which of the following is an unexpected finding and may indicate pathology?
   a. Kyphosis
   b. Cognitive changes
   c. Dyspnea on exertion or stress
   d. Decrease in deep tendon reflexes

2. The physician prescribes nonsteroidal anti-inflammatory drugs (NSAIDs) for an older client with degenerative arthritis. Because of the side effects of NSAIDs, the nurse will teach the client and family to monitor for
   a. pruritus.
   b. fluid retention.
   c. muscle weakness.
   d. gastrointestinal distress.

3. The most common endocrine disorder in the older client is
   a. hypothyroidism.
   b. diabetes mellitus.
   c. Cushing's disease.
   d. diabetes insipidus.

4. An older client has been admitted to an acute care setting following a fracture of the hip. To prevent friction and shearing damage to the skin of this client, the nursing assistants are instructed to
   a. use plastic or rubber sheet protectors.
   b. monitor for nutrition and weight loss.
   c. use a turning sheet for positioning in the bed.
   d. keep the head of the bed elevated 45°.

5. Which of the following is a correct statement about the financing of elder care?
   a. Medicare does not pay for hearing aids, prescription drugs, or glasses.
   b. Routine medical checkups and health screening tests are covered by Medicare.
   c. Medicaid was developed to pay for long-term care for most Americans after age 65.
   d. Costs for elder care have been generally stable since the Balanced Budget Act of 1997.

Rehabilitation, Home Health, Long-Term Care, and Hospice

Key Terms

Match the following terms with their correct definitions.

___ 1. Accreditation

___ 2. Adult Day Care

___ 3. Assisted Living

___ 4. Certification

___ 5. Hospice

___ 6. Licensure

___ 7. Long-Term Care Facility

___ 8. Medicaid

___ 9. Medicare

___10. Medigap Insurance

___11. Rehabilitation

a. Insurance plan for people with Medicare that pays for health care costs not covered by Medicare.

b. Voluntary process that establishes and evaluates compliance with rules and regulations; mandatory for any health care services receiving federal funds.

c. Process by which a voluntary, nongovernmental agency or organization appraises and grants accredited status to institutions and/or programs or services that meet predetermined structure, process, and outcome criteria.

d. Government title program (XIX) that pays for health services for the aged, poor, disabled, and low-income families with dependent children.

e. Mandatory system of granting licenses according to specified standards.

f. Process designed to assist individuals to reach their optimal level of physical, mental, and psychosocial functioning.

g. Care and service that provides a break to caregivers and is utilized for a few hours a week, for an occasional weekend, or for longer periods of time.

h. Abnormal pattern of movement that results from an overactive stretch reflex due to central nervous system damage.

i. Humane, compassionate care provided to clients who can no longer benefit from curative treatment, and have 6 months or less to live.

j. Combination of housing and services for people who require assistance with activities of daily living.

k. Health care facility that provides services to individuals who are not acutely ill, have continuing health care needs, and cannot function independently at home.

___12. Respite Care

l. Provision of a variety of services in a protective setting for adults who are unable to stay alone, but who do not need 24-hour care.

___13. Subacute Care

m. Amendment (Title XVII) to the Social Security act that helps finance the health care of people over 65 years old and of permanently disabled younger people who receive Social Security disability benefits.

___14. Synergy

n. Health care designed to provide services for clients who are out of the acute stage of illness but who still require skilled nursing, monitoring, and ongoing treatments.

Abbreviation Review

Write the definition of the following acronyms.

1. AHCA _____
2. ALFA _____
3. CARF _____
4. CCRC _____
5. CEPN-LTC™ _____
6. CHAP _____
7. CLTC _____
8. ECF _____
9. HCFA _____
10. HMO _____
11. IADL _____
12. ICF _____
13. IHCT _____
14. JCAHO _____
15. NCSBN _____
16. OBRA _____
17. SNF _____

Exercises and Activities

1. Explain factors that have led to an increased use of nonacute health care services.

_____
_____
_____
_____

a. Identify components of the Omnibus Budget Reconciliation Act (OBRA) related to long-term care facilities.

_____

_____

_____

b. List several "rights" provided by the resident's rights document that directly affect your nursing care of clients in long-term care facilities.

(1) _____

(2) _____

(3) _____

(4) _____

(5) _____

(6) _____

c. How would you compare Medicare and Medicaid for the type of assistance they provide?

_____

_____

_____

2. Describe the goal of rehabilitation for the client. When does rehabilitation begin?

_____

_____

_____

a. What skills are important for the nurse working in the field of rehabilitation?

_____

_____

_____

b. Identify services that might be used in home health care for the client or family.

_____

_____

_____

c. What are the nurse's responsibilities in the home health care setting?

_____

_____

_____

3. Compare each of the following types of assistance for clients.

Extended-care facility: _____

_____

Subacute care: _____

_____

Assisted living: _____

_____

Respite care: _____

_____

Adult day care: _____

_____

4. Thomas Patterson is a 38-year-old insurance agent who enjoys writing short stories as a hobby. Last week during a storm, a car coming toward him crossed into his lane, hitting him head-on. The driver in a van following his car saw the accident but was unable to stop, causing a second collision. Mr. Patterson was tossed around in the car and thrown out through the windshield. Rescue workers arrived and transported him to the trauma center. After stabilization of the injury and further assessment, it was determined Mr. Patterson had sustained a T8 injury and is paraplegic. Next week he will be transferred to a rehabilitation facility with a spinal cord injury program. An interdisciplinary health care team (IHCT) will focus on assisting Mr. Patterson to regain as much independence as possible.

   a. Describe the importance of the IHCT for this client in rehabilitation.

   _____

   _____

   _____

   _____

   b. How will the nurse function as a member of this team?

   _____

   _____

   _____

   _____

   c. Why is the early assessment and intervention of psychological well-being essential in the rehabilitation process?

   _____

   _____

   _____

   _____

   d. How can the nurse and the IHCT support Mr. Patterson's efforts toward independence?

   _____

   _____

   _____

   _____

e. One month after his transfer, Mr. Patterson appears to be doing well. He has some function of his upper body, including his hands. His immediate learning needs are AM care, feeding and grooming, intermittent self-catheterization, and bowel training. List several long-term goals for this client.

(1) _____

(2) _____

(3) _____

(4) _____

(5) _____

f. Why will good nutrition and skin care be lifelong issues for this client?

_____

_____

_____

_____

g. Mr. Patterson has limited insurance coverage for the rehabilitation facility. He is now being discharged home and will be seen as an outpatient for 3 hours a day. Mr. Patterson is divorced, and will be moving into his parents' home at least until he has completed his rehabilitation program. How can home health support his transition to independence?

_____

_____

_____

_____

_____

_____

Self-Assessment Questions

Circle the letter that corresponds to the best answer for each question.

1. For the client with a terminal illness, hospice may be utilized for
   a. rehabilitation.
   b. assisted living.
   c. palliative care.
   d. long-term care.

2. A home health nurse has been assigned to care for a client with a chronic illness following discharge from the hospital. A major priority for this nurse will be to
   a. educate the client and family.
   b. maintain accurate documentation.
   c. obtain Medicare/Medicaid funding.
   d. determine the most appropriate placement for long-term care.

3. A primary effect of the Omnibus Budget Reconciliation Act of 1987 on long-term care (LTC) was to
   a. determine funding for LTC facilities.
   b. regulate the reporting of client abuse.
   c. provide accreditation for LTC facilities.
   d. develop the resident's rights document.

4. The increase in nonacute health care services over the past 10 years is related to all but which of the following factors?
   a. Change in costs of health care
   b. Decline in hospital-bed availability
   c. Longer life span of clients with health problems
   d. Early discharge of clients from acute care settings

5. A 68-year-old widowed client, who has just had abdominal surgery for cancer, is expected to do well. There are no family members able to care for the client following early discharge. The most appropriate short-term placement for this client is
   a. hospice.
   b. respite care.
   c. subacute care.
   d. assisted living.

Nursing Care of the Client: Responding to Emergencies

Key Terms

Match the following terms with their correct definitions.

___ 1. Chain of Custody

___ 2. Emergency

___ 3. Emergency Medical Technician

___ 4. Emergency Nursing

___ 5. Glasgow Coma Scale

___ 6. Paramedic

___ 7. Shock

___ 8. Trauma

___ 9. Triage

a. Medical or surgical condition requiring immediate or timely intervention to prevent permanent disability or death.

b. Neurological screening test that measures a client's best verbal, motor, and eye response to stimuli.

c. Documentation of the transfer of evidence (of a crime) from one worker to the next in a secure fashion.

d. Condition of profound hemodynamic and metabolic disturbance characterized by inadequate tissue perfusion and inadequate circulation to the vital organs.

e. Classification of clients to determine priority of need and proper place of treatment.

f. Health care professional trained to provide basic life-saving measures prior to arrival at the hospital.

g. Specialized health care professional trained to provide advanced life support to the client requiring emergency interventions.

h. Care of clients who require emergency interventions.

i. Wound or injury.

Abbreviation Review

Write the definition of the following abbreviations and acronyms.

1. ABC _____

2. cc _____

3. cm _____

4. CPR _____

5. ED _____

6. EMS _____

7. EMT _____

8. EMT-P _____

9. MVA_____

10. RICE _____

Exercises and Activities

1. Describe the role of the nurse in emergency care.

   _____

   _____

   _____

   _____

   a. List the "golden rules" of emergency care or first aid.

   (1) _____   (5) _____

   (2) _____   (6) _____

   (3) _____   (7) _____

   (4) _____

   b. Why do hospitals and emergency care organizations use triage systems for evaluating clients?

   _____

   _____

   _____

   c. How does the Good Samaritan Law protect the client and the caregiver?

   _____

   _____

   _____

2. Identify two common causes for each type of shock.

   Hypovolemic: Anaphylactic:

   (1) _____   (1) _____

   (2) _____   (2) _____

   Cardiogenic: Neurogenic:

   (1) _____   (1) _____

   (2) _____   (2) _____

   Septic:

   (1) _____

   (2) _____

   a. How can the nurse assess the neurological status of a client?

   _____

   _____

   _____

3. Compare the medical treatment and at least three nursing interventions for each of the following categories of emergencies.

	Medical Treatment	*Nursing Interventions*
Abdominal	(1) (2) (3)	
Cardiopulmonary	(1) (2) (3)	
Musculoskeletal	(1) (2) (3)	
Neurological	(1) (2) (3)	

a. Describe the immediate care for the client with an ocular injury.

_____

_____

_____

b. Following examination and x-rays, a client is diagnosed with a sprain to the right ankle. How would you explain the "RICE" treatment for this client to use at home?

_____

_____

_____

c. Identify the special needs of sexual assault victims. What tests and medications may be included in their care?

_____

_____

_____

_____

4. Mrs. Levinson, a 73-year-old grandparent, had joined her son, daughter-in-law, and two of their children for a day at their county fair and music festival. Although she was drinking what she thought was adequate fluid, as the afternoon continued Mrs. Levinson developed a headache, mild weakness, and nausea. She was sure the feelings would pass with a short rest. However, she soon developed symptoms of heat stroke and was transported to the community hospital 5 miles away.

   a. Compare signs and symptoms for heat cramps, heat exhaustion, and heat stroke.

      _____

      _____

      _____

   b. What subjective and objective data would be collected on admission to the emergency facility?

      _____

      _____

      _____

   c. Describe immediate medical and pharmacological treatment that would be used with Mrs. Levinson.

      _____

      _____

      _____

   d. Identify nursing interventions that would be appropriate for this client.

      (1) _____

      (2) _____

      (3) _____

      (4) _____

      (5) _____

   e. A medication that Mrs. Levinson had been using for a short time had contributed to her susceptibility to heat injury. What precautions could you suggest for her to prevent heat injury in the future?

      _____

      _____

      _____

      _____

      _____

Self-Assessment Questions

Circle the letter that corresponds to the best answer for each question.

  1. A client arrives at a busy emergency room with a compound fracture of the right leg. Using the principles of hospital triage, the nurse assesses this condition as
    a. urgent.
    b. emergent.
    c. nonurgent.
    d. life threatening.

2. A client arrives in the emergency room with active bleeding from an abdominal wound and multiple leg wounds. Assessment indicates the client is in shock. The first priority for the health care team will be to
   a. notify the next of kin.
   b. determine the precipitating events.
   c. control active bleeding as quickly as possible.
   d. determine if airway and breathing are adequate.

3. A client is brought into the emergency room after falling from a roof. Because a spinal cord injury is suspected, this client is at risk for
   a. traumatic shock.
   b. neurogenic shock.
   c. cardiogenic shock.
   d. anaphylactic shock.

4. Late signs of increased intracranial pressure include dilated pupils, widened pulse pressure, spontaneous emesis, and
   a. tremors.
   b. dyspnea.
   c. headache.
   d. hiccoughs.

5. Emergency personnel arrive at the scene of a two-car accident on the shoulder of a busy interstate highway. One car has a victim who appears trapped inside and unconscious. The first priority for the emergency personnel will be to
   a. ensure their own safety.
   b. call for additional help if needed.
   c. remove the victim from immediate danger.
   d. determine whether the injuries are life threatening.

6. The client arrives at the emergency room with a neighbor following a bee sting. Assessment findings include edema in the throat, difficulty breathing, hypotension, and tachycardia. Medical treatment for this client will most likely include
   a. digoxin.
   b. epinephrine.
   c. fluid replacement.
   d. a broad-spectrum antibiotic.

Critical Thinking on Multiple Systems

Exercises and Activities

1. Why is critical thinking important in discovering the relationship between disease process and symptoms?

   _____

   _____

   _____

   _____

   _____

   a. How will critical thinking help you to set priorities for nursing care?

   _____

   _____

   _____

   _____

   _____

2. Your facility has initiated a policy of evaluating a client's level of pain on a frequent, routine basis. In what ways can chronic or uncontrolled pain affect the client? Give specific examples of how pain affects several systems.

   _____

   _____

   _____

   _____

   _____

3. Identify at least four systems that may be affected by each of the following diseases.

Sickle cell anemia	(1) _____	(3) _____
	(2) _____	(4) _____
COPD	(1) _____	(3) _____
	(2) _____	(4) _____
Graves' disease	(1) _____	(3) _____
	(2) _____	(4) _____

4. One of your clients, Mr. Fogel, was diagnosed with multiple sclerosis 9 years ago and has symptoms that flare up at frequent intervals. He tried living alone, but moved in with his brother who has provided some care for the past two years. Mr. Fogel has been admitted to your unit with dehydration and a urinary tract infection. However, he is also experiencing blurred vision, tremors, and vertigo. Walking without assistance is nearly impossible for him. You note that your client appears pale, older than his stated age, and underweight with muscle atrophy. He appears somewhat depressed.

   a. How is a client diagnosed with multiple sclerosis?

   _____
   _____
   _____
   _____
   _____

   b. Describe the pathophysiology of this disease.

   _____
   _____
   _____
   _____
   _____

   c. Identify the systems that are often affected.

   _____
   _____
   _____
   _____
   _____

   d. Select three of the systems associated with his current condition and write the name of each at the top of a column. Below each one, identify manifestations related to that system.

e. Develop a care plan for Mr. Fogel based on his current needs. Determine which diagnoses have the greatest priority.

Nursing Diagnoses	Goals	Interventions
(1)		
(2)		
(3)		

f. After several days of treatment for a UTI and weight loss, including antibiotics, intravenous fluids, and nutrition support, Mr. Fogel will be discharged home with his brother. What items do you think will be most important to emphasize in your discharge teaching and why?

_____

_____

_____

_____

_____

5. Mrs. Myers, a client on your skilled nursing unit, is 87 years old. She was an elementary school teacher and community activist for many years. She has one son who lives several hours away. Mrs. Myers was hospitalized after she had apparently suffered a serious left side CVA (stroke) at her retirement community. Mrs. Myers will stay in your skilled care unit until her son can arrange for admission to a facility closer to his home.

a. What signs and symptoms might you note in your client?

_____

_____

_____

_____

_____

b. Why would Mrs. Myers exhibit different signs and symptoms if she had a right side CVA?

_____

_____

_____

_____

c. Why might antihypertensive medications and thrombolytic agents be administered?

_____

_____

_____

_____

d. Why might Mrs. Fogel be placed on fluid restriction?

_____

_____

_____

_____

e. Select three systems that a CVA can affect and write one in each column. Below each, list manifestations associated with those systems.

f. Mrs. Myers is recovering now but will need almost total assistance for ADLs. You note that she needs help with eating, bathing, and ROM exercises, and needs meticulous skin care. She still appears confused and is having trouble speaking. Physical assessment, vital signs, medication administration, and rehabilitation activities are also included in your plan of care for today. The previous set of vital signs showed Mrs. Myers's blood pressure was elevated. Which nursing interventions will you give the highest priority and why? Can you safely delegate any activities to a nursing assistant (UAP)?

_____

_____

_____

_____

Answer Key

Chapter 1 The Health Care Delivery System

Key Terms

1. d
2. a
3. e
4. j
5. o
6. i
7. b
8. k
9. p
10. l
11. c
12. f
13. n
14. g
15. m
16. h
17. q
18. r

Abbreviation Review

1. Alcohol, Drug Abuse, and Mental Health Administration
2. Agency for Health Care Policy and Research
3. acquired immunodeficiency syndrome
4. American Medical Association
5. American Nurses Association
6. advanced practice registered nurse
7. Agency for Toxic Substances and Disease Registry
8. coronary care unit
9. Centers for Disease Control and Prevention
10. Children's Health Insurance Program
11. certified nurse midwife
12. community nursing organization
13. clinical nurse specialist
14. computed tomography
15. doctor of dental surgery
16. doctor of dental medicine
17. diagnosis-related group
18. electrocardiogram
19. emergency department
20. electroencephalograph
21. electromyogram
22. exclusive provider organization
23. Food and Drug Administration
24. Health Care Financing Administration
25. human immunodeficiency virus
26. health maintenance organization
27. Health Resources and Services Administration
28. intensive care unit
29. Indian Health Service
30. Joint Commission on the Accreditation of Healthcare Organizations
31. licensed practical/vocational nurse
32. medical doctor
33. magnetic resonance imaging
34. National Council of State Boards of Nursing
35. National Federation of Licensed Practical Nurses
36. National Institutes of Health
37. National League for Nursing
38. nurse practitioner
39. operating room
40. occupational therapist
41. physician's assistant
42. primary care provider
43. preferred provider organization
44. physical therapist
45. registered dietitian
46. registered nurse
47. rural primary care hospital

48. registered pharmacist
49. recovery room
50. respiratory therapist
51. school-based clinic
52. social worker
53. U.S. Department of Health and Human Services
54. U.S. Public Health Service
55. Veterans Administration

Self-Assessment Questions

1. a
2. c
3. b
4. a
5. a
6. c

Chapter 2   Critical Thinking

Key Terms

1. f
2. c
3. d
4. g
5. j
6. a
7. h
8. k
9. b
10. i
11. e

Abbreviation Review

1. Universal Intellectual Standards

Self-Assessment Questions

1. b
2. a
3. d
4. a
5. c
6. d
7. d

Chapter 3   Legal Responsibilities

Key Terms

1. d
2. g
3. n
4. t
5. x
6. cc
7. hh
8. m
9. u
10. ee
11. c
12. w
13. h
14. v
15. o
16. b
17. l
18. dd
19. e
20. q
21. p
22. gg
23. f
24. bb
25. kk
26. i
27. y
28. jj
29. j
30. ff
31. ll
32. r
33. ii
34. z
35. s
36. aa
37. a
38. k

Abbreviation Review

1. American Dietetic Association
2. Americans with Disabilities Act
3. against medical advice

4. American Medical Association

5. American Nurses Association

6. cardiopulmonary resuscitation

7. do not resuscitate

8. durable power of attorney for health care

9. human immunodeficiency virus

10. intramuscular

11. Joint Commission on Accreditation of Healthcare Organizations

12. licensed practical/vocational nurse

13. National Council Licensure Exam

14. National Federation of Licensed Practical Nurses

15. *nil per os,* Latin for "nothing by mouth"

16. *per os,* Latin for "by mouth"

17. registered nurse

Self-Assessment Questions

1. c
2. d
3. b
4. a
5. b

Chapter 4   Ethical Responsibilities

Key Terms

1. i
2. m
3. q
4. n
5. b
6. h
7. l
8. r
9. f
10. t
11. c
12. j
13. u
14. x
15. k
16. v
17. y
18. w

19. g
20. p
21. a
22. d
23. o
24. s
25. e

Abbreviation Review

1. American Hospital Association

2. American Nurses Association

3. International Council of Nurses

4. licensed practical/vocational nurse

5. National Federation of Licensed Practical Nurses

6. Veterans Affairs, Veterans Administration

Self-Assessment Questions

1. d
2. a
3. b
4. a
5. c
6. b

Chapter 5   Communication

Key Terms

1. e
2. n
3. k
4. o
5. c
6. j
7. p
8. d
9. m
10. h
11. b
12. l
13. i
14. f
15. a
16. g

Abbreviation Review

1. computerized patient record
2. human immunodeficiency virus
3. Institute of Medicine
4. licensed practical/vocational nurse
5. registered nurse
6. words per minute

Self-Assessment Questions

1. a
2. b
3. b
4. d
5. a
6. d

Chapter 6   Cultural Diversity and Nursing

Key Terms

1. d
2. j
3. n
4. e
5. k
6. f
7. o
8. c
9. g
10. l
11. h
12. p
13. b
14. i
15. m
16. q
17. a

Abbreviation Review

1. World Health Organization

Self-Assessment Questions

1. c
2. a
3. b

4. c
5. b

Chapter 7   Wellness Concepts

Key Terms

1. c
2. d
3. f
4. a
5. e
6. b

Abbreviation Review

1. acquired immunodeficiency syndrome
2. Centers for Disease Control and Prevention
3. electrocardiogram
4. electrocardiogram
5. hemoglobin
6. human immunodeficiency virus
7. low density lipoprotein
8. papanicolau test
9. red blood cell, red blood count
10. sun protection factor
11. U.S. Department of Health and Human Services
12. World Health Organization

Self-Assessment Questions

1. c
2. b
3. a
4. b
5. c

Chapter 8   Alternative/Complementary Therapies

Key Terms

1. f
2. n
3. d
4. y
5. m
6. g

7. o

8. s

9. k

10. a

11. z

12. t

13. aa

14. h

15. b

16. j

17. l

18. i

19. p

20. v

21. e

22. q

23. c

24. x

25. r

26. u

27. w

Abbreviation Review

1. American Holistic Nurses' Association

2. Food and Drug Administration

3. low-density lipoprotein

4. National Center for Complementary and Alternative Medicine

5. Office of Alternative Medicine

6. progressive muscle relaxation

7. psychoneuroimmunology

Self-Assessment Questions

1. a

2. d

3. a

4. b

5. d

6. c

7. c

Chapter 9   Loss, Grief, and Death

Key Terms

1. i

2. m

3. v

4. f

5. p

6. a

7. j

8. w

9. q

10. b

11. aa

12. c

13. r

14. x

15. d

16. k

17. u

18. e

19. l

20. z

21. n

22. g

23. s

24. o

25. h

26. y

27. t

Abbreviation Review

1. American Nurses Association

2. do not resuscitate

3. health maintenance organization

4. intramuscular

5. morphine sulfate

6. North American Nursing Diagnosis Association

7. Omnibus Budget Reconciliation Act

8. Patient Self-Determination Act

9. posttraumatic stress disorder

10. sudden infant death syndrome

Self-Assessment Questions

1. c

2. b

3. c

4. d

5. c

Chapter 10   Fluid, Electrolyte, and Acid–Base Balance

Key Terms

1. oo
2. t
3. cc
4. pp
5. e
6. dd
7. s
8. f
9. bb
10. qq
11. g
12. rr
13. h
14. r
15. u
16. ee
17. v
18. tt
19. kk
20. gg
21. n
22. m
23. b
24. ss
25. ff
26. a
27. i
28. p
29. w
30. ll
31. o
32. uu
33. c
34. x
35. aa
36. d
37. mm
38. q
39. z
40. hh
41. j
42. ii
43. nn
44. y
45. k
46. jj
47. l

Abbreviation Review

1. arterial blood gases
2. antidiuretic hormone
3. adenosine triphosphatase
4. blood urea nitrogen
5. calcium ion
6. calcium chloride
7. chloride ion
8. carbon dioxide ion
9. carboxyl group
10. dextrose 5% in water
11. deciliter
12. extracellular fluid
13. hydrogen ion
14. carbonic acid
15. water
16. hydrochloric acid
17. bicarbonate ion
18. hematocrit
19. hemoglobin
20. intake and output
21. intracellular fluid
22. potassium ion
23. potassium chloride
24. kilogram
25. liter
26. pound
27. milliequivalent
28. milligram
29. magnesium ion
30. magnesium chloride
31. milliliter
32. millimeters of mercury
33. Milk of Magnesia
34. milliosmoles/kilogram
35. sodium ion

36. disodium phosphate
37. sodium sulfate
38. sodium chloride
39. sodium dihydrogen phosphate
40. sodium bicarbonate
41. sodium monohydrogen phosphate
42. sodium hydroxide
43. amino group
44. oxygen
45. hydroxyl
46. partial pressure of carbon dioxide
47. potential hydrogen
48. partial pressure of oxygen
49. phosphate ion
50. oxygen saturation
51. total parenteral nutrition
52. temperature, pulse, respirations
53. weight

Self-Assessment Questions

1. d
2. a
3. b
4. a
5. c
6. a
7. b

Chapter 11   IV Therapy

Key Terms

1. h
2. g
3. k
4. n
5. l
6. f
7. a
8. b
9. i
10. m
11. d
12. j
13. c
14. e

Abbreviation Review

1. central venous catheter
2. dextrose 5% in water
3. intravenous
4. intravenous piggyback
5. keep vein open
6. liter
7. milliliter
8. peripheral intravenous
9. vascular access device

Self-Assessment Questions

1. c
2. b
3. c
4. d
5. b

Chapter 12   Health Assessment

Key Terms

1. i
2. u
3. l
4. a
5. m
6. v
7. dd
8. s
9. j
10. d
11. cc
12. t
13. k
14. ff
15. z
16. w
17. ee
18. b
19. n
20. f
21. bb
22. o
23. e
24. p
25. r

26. y
27. q
28. h
29. c
30. x
31. g
32. aa

Abbreviation Review

1. apical pulse
2. blood pressure
3. centimeter
4. left lower quadrant
5. level of consciousness
6. left upper quadrant
7. pulse
8. pupils equal, round, reactive to light and accommodation
9. respiration
10. right lower quadrant
11. review of systems
12. right upper quadrant
13. temperature

Self-Assessment Questions

1. b
2. c
3. d
4. a
5. c
6. b

Chapter 13   Diagnostic Tests

Key Terms

1. l
2. x
3. k
4. vv
5. ll
6. a
7. uu
8. m
9. n
10. xx
11. jj
12. y
13. tt
14. d
15. o
16. kk
17. e
18. ff
19. i
20. w
21. mm
22. rr
23. j
24. nn
25. ww
26. pp
27. b
28. ii
29. c
30. aa
31. p
32. ss
33. q
34. ccc
35. z
36. gg
37. ee
38. h
39. u
40. dd
41. v
42. yy
43. hh
44. g
45. t
46. cc
47. zz
48. bbb
49. s
50. oo
51. aaa
52. f
53. bb
54. qq
55. r

Abbreviation Review

1. arterial blood gas
2. culture and sensitivity
3. cerebrospinal fluid
4. computed tomography
5. electrocardiogram
6. electroencephalogram
7. human immunodeficiency virus
8. intake and output
9. intravenous
10. intravenous pyelogram
11. partial pressure of carbon dioxide
12. partial pressure of oxygen
13. red blood cell, red blood count
14. white blood cell, white blood count

Self-Assessment Questions

1. c
2. a
3. b
4. d
5. c
6. d

Chapter 14   Pain Management

Key Terms

1. hh
2. a
3. g
4. bb
5. aa
6. ii
7. rr
8. kk
9. b
10. gg
11. jj
12. h
13. y
14. j
15. c
16. z
17. i
18. ll

19. k
20. cc
21. t
22. f
23. o
24. mm
25. p
26. dd
27. n
28. e
29. u
30. ff
31. v
32. d
33. m
34. w
35. l
36. x
37. oo
38. qq
39. ee
40. s
41. r
42. q
43. nn
44. pp

Abbreviation Review

1. American Pain Society
2. Agency for Health Care Policy and Research
3. around the clock
4. eutectic (cream) mixture of local anesthetics
5. hydrochloric acid
6. International Association for the Study of Pain
7. microgram
8. magnetic resonance imaging
9. *nil per os,* Latin for "nothing by mouth"
10. nonsteroidal anti-inflammatory drug
11. patient-controlled analgesia
12. *per os,* Latin for "by mouth"
13. *pro re nata,* Latin for "as required"
14. every

15. subcutaneous
16. tetracaine, adrenaline, cocaine
17. transcutaneous electrical nerve stimulation
18. temporomandibular joint
19. Visual Analog Scale
20. World Health Organization

Self-Assessment Questions

1. a
2. b
3. b
4. c
5. d

Chapter 15   Anesthesia

Key Terms

1. b
2. g
3. i
4. h
5. f
6. a
7. d
8. c
9. j
10. e

Abbreviation Review

1. cubic centimeter
2. central nervous system
3. certified registered nurse anesthetist
4. cerebrospinal fluid
5. endotracheal tube
6. heart rate
7. nonsteroidal anti-inflammatory drug
8. patient-controlled analgesia
9. postdural puncture headache

Self-Assessment Questions

1. d
2. b
3. b
4. a
5. d
6. b

Chapter 16   Nursing Care of the Surgical Client

Key Terms

1. l
2. g
3. r
4. o
5. d
6. i
7. n
8. a
9. j
10. b
11. m
12. c
13. p
14. f
15. k
16. q
17. e
18. h

Abbreviation Review

1. alanine aminotransferase
2. Association of Operating Room Nurses
3. aspartate aminotransferase
4. blood urea nitrogen
5. Certified Registered Nurse Anesthetist
6. doctor of osteopathy
7. eyes, ears, nose, and throat
8. electrical surgical unit
9. endotracheal
10. hematocrit
11. hemoglobin
12. liter
13. monamine oxidase
14. milliliter
15. doctor of medicine
16. operating room
17. postanesthesia care unit
18. prothrombin time
19. partial thromboplastin time
20. registered nurse first assistant

Self-Assessment Questions

1. a
2. c
3. d
4. b
5. d
6. a
7. d
8. b

Chapter 17   Nursing Care of the Oncology Client

Key Terms

1. h
2. d
3. q
4. g
5. p
6. a
7. i
8. w
9. r
10. o
11. e
12. j
13. n
14. f
15. b
16. s
17. k
18. m
19. v
20. t
21. x
22. l
23. y
24. z
25. u
26. c

Abbreviation Review

1. American Cancer Society
2. Agency for Health Care Policy and Research
3. *bacillus Calmette-Guérin*
4. bone marrow transplantation
5. cell-cycle nonspecific
6. cell-cycle specific
7. central nervous system
8. computed tomography
9. deoxyribonucleic acid
10. Environmental Protection Agency
11. explantable venous access device
12. implantable vascular access device
13. Occupational Safety and Health Administration
14. ribonucleic acid
15. transcutaneous electrical nerve stimulation
16. tumor, node, metastasis
17. total parenteral nutrition

Self-Assessment Questions

1. c
2. b
3. b
4. d
5. c

Chapter 18   Nursing Care of the Client: Respiratory System

Key Terms

1. g
2. e
3. w
4. x
5. gg
6. m
7. y
8. l
9. z
10. aa
11. f
12. bb
13. hh
14. a
15. cc
16. n
17. dd

18. jj
19. b
20. o
21. q
22. v
23. ff
24. i
25. u
26. t
27. h
28. d
29. s
30. j
31. ee
32. r
33. c
34. kk
35. k
36. p
37. ii

Abbreviation Review

1. arterial blood gas
2. acid-fast bacillus
3. activated partial thromboplastin time
4. adult respiratory distress syndrome
5. antireptolysin O
6. *bacillus Calmette-Guérin*
7. chronic airflow limitation
8. computerized axial tomography
9. congestive heart failure
10. carbon dioxide
11. chronic obstructive lung disease
12. chronic obstructive pulmonary disease
13. computed tomography
14. cerebrovascular accident
15. hydrogen ion
16. carbonic acid
17. bicarbonate ion
18. Isoniazid
19. international normalized ratio
20. intravenous
21. liter
22. milliequivalents per liter
23. minute
24. cubic millimeter

25. magnetic resonance imaging
26. nonsteroidal anti-inflammatory drug
27. partial pressure of carbon dioxide
28. partial pressure of oxygen
29. pulmonary function test
30. potential hydrogen
31. purified protein derivative
32. prothrombin time
33. oxygen saturation
34. tuberculosis

Self-Assessment Questions

1. d
2. b
3. d
4. c
5. b
6. c

Chapter 19   Nursing Care of the Client: Cardiovascular System

Key Terms

1. k
2. oo
3. aa
4. nn
5. l
6. mm
7. ll
8. m
9. z
10. aaa
11. kk
12. uu
13. n
14. y
15. a
16. jj
17. o
18. x
19. b
20. p
21. w
22. hh
23. c

24. v
25. ii
26. s
27. j
28. bb
29. d
30. i
31. r
32. cc
33. e
34. q
35. yy
36. pp
37. f
38. zz
39. dd
40. gg
41. t
42. g
43. ee
44. u
45. ff
46. h
47. qq
48. tt
49. xx
50. ww
51. rr
52. vv
53. ss

Abbreviation Review

1. abdominal aortic aneurysm
2. angiotensin-converting enzyme
3. automatic implantable cardioverter-defibrillator
4. antilymphocytic globulin
5. activated partial thromboplastin time
6. aspartate aminotransferase
7. antihymocytic globulin
8. atrioventricular
9. coronary artery bypass graft
10. coronary artery disease
11. coronary artery heart disease
12. complete blood count
13. congestive heart failure
14. creatine kinase or creatine phosphokinase
15. cardiopulmonary resuscitation
16. deep vein thrombosis
17. electrocardiogram
18. erythrocyte sedimentation rate
19. hematocrit
20. high density lipoprotein
21. hemoglobin
22. hypertension
23. intra-aortic balloon pump
24. intensive care unit
25. International Normalized Ratio
26. lactic dehydrogenase
27. low density lipoprotein
28. myocardial infarction
29. magnetic resonance imaging
30. multigated acquisition
31. premature atrial contraction
32. paroxysmal atrial tachycardia
33. paroxysmal supraventricular tachycardia
34. prothrombin time
35. percutaneous transluminal coronary angioplasty
36. partial thromboplastin time
37. sinoatrial
38. serum glutamate oxaloacetate transaminase
39. transesophageal echocardiography
40. ventricular assist device
41. ventricular fibrillation
42. very low-density lipoprotein
43. ventricular tachycardia

Self-Assessment Questions

1. b
2. c
3. a
4. b
5. d
6. a
7. d

Chapter 20   Nursing Care of the Client: Hematologic and Lymphatic Systems

Key Terms

1. c
2. h
3. o
4. b
5. i
6. k
7. a
8. n
9. j
10. p
11. y
12. g
13. q
14. x
15. f
16. l
17. v
18. m
19. t
20. w
21. e
22. u
23. r
24. s
25. d

Abbreviation Review

1. a combination of chemotherapy drugs: doxorubicin (Adriamycin), bleomycin sulfate (Blenoxane), vinblastine (Velban), dacarbazine (DTIC-Dome)
2. acute lymphocytic leukemia
3. acute myelocytic leukemia
4. antithymocyte globulin
5. a combination of chemotherapy drugs: cyclophosphamide (Cytoxan), doxorubicin (Adriamycin), vincristine (Oncovin), prednisone (Deltasone)
6. chronic lymphocytic leukemia
7. chronic myelocytic leukemia
8. a combination of chemotherapy drugs: cyclophosphamide (Cytoxan), vincristine (Oncovin), procarbazine (Matulanel), prednisone (Deltasone)
9. a combination of chemotherapy drugs: cyclophosphamide (Cytoxan), vincristine (Oncovin), prednisone (Deltasone)
10. disseminated intravascular coagulation
11. hematocrit
12. Hodgkin's disease
13. hemoglobin
14. human leukocyte antigen
15. idiopathic thrombocytopenic purpura
16. lactic dehydrogenase
17. a combination of chemotherapy drugs: mechlorethamine or nitrogen mustard (Mustargen), vincristine (Oncovin), procarbazine hydrochloride (Matulane), prednisone (Deltasone)
18. non-Hodgkin's lymphoma
19. patient-controlled analgesia
20. polymorphonuclear leukocyte
21. prothrombin time
22. partial thromboplastin time
23. red blood cell
24. total iron binding capacity
25. white blood cell

Self-Assessment Questions

1. c
2. b
3. c
4. a
5. d
6. a

Chapter 21   Nursing Care of the Client: Integumentary System

Key Terms

1. e
2. n
3. t
4. u
5. o
6. d

7. m
8. v
9. cc
10. s
11. gg
12. dd
13. b
14. f
15. w
16. l
17. i
18. r
19. p
20. x
21. bb
22. ee
23. a
24. c
25. g
26. y
27. k
28. aa
29. h
30. ff
31. hh
32. q
33. z
34. j

Abbreviation Review

1. asymmetry, border, color, diameter
2. angiogenesis factor
3. fibroblast activating factor
4. methicillin-resistant *Staphylococcus aureus*
5. National Pressure Ulcer Advisory Panel
6. psorafen ultraviolet A-range
7. range of motion
8. sun protection factor
9. U.S. Department of Health and Human Services
10. vacuum-assisted closure

Self-Assessment Questions

1. a
2. b

3. a
4. c
5. a
6. d
7. c

Chapter 22   Nursing Care of the Client: Immune System

Key Terms

1. d
2. e
3. n
4. p
5. u
6. c
7. h
8. a
9. o
10. v
11. i
12. w
13. x
14. q
15. b
16. j
17. e
18. m
19. s
20. f
21. k
22. r
23. t
24. l

Abbreviation Review

1. American College of Rheumatology
2. antinuclear antibody
3. computed tomography
4. disease-modifying anti-rheumatic drug
5. deoxyribonucleic acid
6. enzyme-linked immunosorbent assay
7. electromyogram
8. erythrocyte sedimentation rate
9. Food and Drug Administration

10. gastrointenstinal
11. immunoglobulin G
12. immunoglobulin M
13. lupus erythematosus
14. myasthenia gravis
15. National Institute of Allergy and Infectious Diseases
16. *nil per os,* Latin for "nothing by mouth"
17. nucleoside analog reverse transcriptase inhibitor
18. rheumatoid arthritis
19. rheumatoid factor
20. range of motion
21. systemic lupus erythematosus
22. sun protection factor

Self-Assessment Questions

1. a
2. c
3. a
4. b
5. c

Chapter 23   Nursing Care of the Client: HIV and AIDS

Key Terms

1. b
2. l
3. e
4. f
5. h
6. a
7. i
8. j
9. d
10. k
11. c
12. g

Abbreviation Review

1. AIDS dementia complex
2. acid-fast bacillus
3. Centers for Disease Control and Prevention

4. cervical intraepithelial neoplasia
5. cytomegalovirus
6. central nervous system
7. enzyme-linked immunosorbent assay
8. hepatitis B virus
9. hepatitis C virus
10. hepatitis D virus
11. human immunodeficiency virus
12. Kaposi's sarcoma
13. *Mycobacterium avium* complex
14. multi-drug-resistant tuberculosis
15. non-Hodgkin's lymphoma
16. National Institutes of Health
17. nonnucleoside reverse transcriptase inhibitor
18. oral hairy leukoplakia
19. Occupational Safety and Health Administration
20. *Pneumocystis carinii* pneumonia
21. polymerase chain reaction
22. purified protein derivative
23. *pro re nata,* Latin for "as needed"
24. ribonucleic acid

Self-Assessment Questions

1. a
2. b
3. c
4. a
5. d

Chapter 24   Nursing Care of the Client: Musculoskeletal System

Key Terms

1. b
2. u
3. i
4. q
5. a
6. v
7. j
8. o
9. c
10. r

11. w
12. k
13. d
14. n
15. h
16. e
17. x
18. l
19. s
20. g
21. t
22. y
23. z
24. m
25. p
26. f

Abbreviation Review

1. bone mineral density
2. circulation movement sensation
3. continuous passive motion
4. degenerative joint disease
5. National Institute of Arthritis and Musculoskeletal and Skin Diseases
6. National Osteoporosis Foundation
7. open reduction/internal fixation
8. rest, ice, compression, and elevation
9. range of motion
10. sequential compression device
11. temporomandibular joint

Self-Assessment Questions

1. a
2. b
3. b
4. d
5. c
6. a

Chapter 25   Nursing Care of the Client: Neurological System

Key Terms

1. z
2. f
3. k

4. q
5. gg
6. aa
7. a
8. dd
9. e
10. r
11. i
12. p
13. qq
14. w
15. d
16. ee
17. ii
18. ll
19. v
20. nn
21. l
22. oo
23. x
24. bb
25. b
26. hh
27. pp
28. kk
29. cc
30. n
31. y
32. jj
33. c
34. mm
35. ff
36. h
37. t
38. o
39. g
40. j
41. m
42. u
43. s

Abbreviation Review

1. adrenocorticotropic hormone
2. Alzheimer's disease
3. amyotrophic lateral sclerosis
4. autonomic nervous system

5. cranial nerve
6. cerebrospinal fluid
7. computerized tomography
8. cerebrovascular accident
9. diffuse axonal injury
10. electroencephalogram
11. γ = aminobutyric acid
12. immunoglobulin
13. monoamine oxidase
14. mean arterial pressure
15. multiple sclerosis
16. monosodium glutamate
17. nonsteroidal anti-inflammatory drug
18. partial pressure of carbon dioxide
19. pupils equal, round, reactive to light and accommodation
20. peripheral nervous system
21. prothrombin time
22. reversible ischemic neurological deficit
23. spinal cord injury
24. transient ischemic attack

Self-Assessment Questions

1. b
2. a
3. c
4. b
5. a

Chapter 26   Nursing Care of the Client: Sensory System

Key Terms

1. qq
2. b
3. z
4. hh
5. r
6. v
7. a
8. cc
9. ii
10. u
11. c
12. q
13. m
14. y
15. p
16. e
17. bb
18. dd
19. n
20. d
21. ll
22. aa
23. jj
24. nn
25. w
26. k
27. ee
28. t
29. j
30. i
31. kk
32. o
33. mm
34. x
35. f
36. g
37. ff
38. s
39. gg
40. l
41. oo
42. pp
43. h

Abbreviation Review

1. autonomic nervous system
2. central nervous system
3. intraocular lens
4. intraocular pressure
5. level of consciousness
6. peripheral nervous system
7. telecommunication device for the deaf
8. University of Pennsylvania Smell Identification Test

Self-Assessment Questions

1. b
2. c
3. d

4. a
5. d
6. c

Chapter 27   Nursing Care of the Client: Endocrine System

Key Terms

1. c
2. m
3. t
4. n
5. a
6. o
7. b
8. e
9. u
10. w
11. l
12. p
13. d
14. v
15. f
16. y
17. h
18. i
19. z
20. bb
21. q
22. g
23. aa
24. x
25. j
26. r
27. k
28. s

Abbreviation Review

1. adrenocorticotropic hormone
2. American Diabetes Association
3. antidiuretic hormone
4. Centers for Disease Control and Prevention
5. cerebrovascular accident
6. diabetic ketoacidosis

7. electrocardiogram
8. follicle-stimulating hormone
9. gestational diabetes mellitus
10. growth hormone
11. hyperosmolar hyperglycemic nonketotic syndrome
12. insulin-dependent diabetes mellitus
13. impaired glucose tolerance
14. intravenous
15. luteinizing hormone
16. melanocyte-stimulating hormone
17. noninsulin-dependent diabetes mellitus
18. parathyroid hormone
19. propylthiouracil
20. peripheral vascular disease
21. thyroid-stimulating hormone

Self-Assessment Questions

1. a
2. b
3. c
4. a
5. c

Chapter 28   Nursing Care of the Client: Gastrointestinal System

Key Terms

1. h
2. w
3. i
4. r
5. x
6. s
7. ee
8. ll
9. kk
10. y
11. j
12. a
13. k
14. z
15. l
16. q
17. b

18. aa
19. p
20. o
21. u
22. ff
23. jj
24. t
25. mm
26. c
27. bb
28. d
29. m
30. gg
31. e
32. cc
33. f
34. v
35. hh
36. dd
37. g
38. n
39. ii

Abbreviation Review

1. alanine aminotransferase
2. aspartate aminotransferase
3. common bile duct
4. carcinoembryonic antigen
5. congestive heart failure
6. esophagogastroduodenoscopy
7. enterostomal
8. gastroesophageal reflux disease
9. gammaglutamy transpeptidase
10. hemoglobin and hematocrit
11. hepatitis A virus
12. hepatitis B immune globulin
13. hydrochloric acid
14. hepatitis C virus
15. hepatitis D virus
16. inflammatory bowel disease
17. lactate dehydrogenase
18. lower esophageal sphincter
19. nasogastric
20. *nil per os,* Latin for "nothing by mouth"
21. nonsteroidal anti-inflammatory drug

22. over-the-counter
23. prothrombin time
24. partial thromboplastin time
25. right lower quadrant
26. transjugular intrahepatic portosystemic shunt
27. ulcerative colitis
28. upper gastrointestinal tract
29. vital signs

Self-Assessment Questions

1. b
2. a
3. b
4. c
5. d
6. c

Chapter 29   Nursing Care of the Client: Urinary System

Key Terms

1. f
2. i
3. r
4. n
5. aa
6. t
7. j
8. e
9. h
10. y
11. k
12. c
13. p
14. g
15. o
16. bb
17. s
18. v
19. q
20. b
21. m

22. w
23. l
24. u
25. a
26. x
27. z
28. d

Abbreviation Review

1. acquired cystic kidney disease
2. American Cancer Society
3. amyotrophic lateral sclerosis
4. acute renal failure
5. acute tubular necrosis
6. arteriovenous
7. benign prostatic hypertrophy
8. culture and sensitivity
9. continuous ambulatory peritoneal dialysis
10. effective arterial blood volume
11. erythrocyte sedimentation rate
12. end-stage renal disease
13. extracorporeal shock wave lithotripsy
14. glomerular filtration rate
15. National Institute of Diabetes and Digestive and Kidney Diseases
16. nonsteroidal anti-inflammatory drug
17. polycystic kidney disease
18. range of motion
19. urinary tract infection

Self-Assessment Questions

1. d
2. b
3. a
4. c
5. a

Chapter 30   Nursing Care of the Client: Female Reproductive System

Key Terms

1. c
2. g
3. l
4. f

5. n
6. a
7. j
8. b
9. h
10. o
11. k
12. p
13. d
14. m
15. q
16. e
17. i

Abbreviation Review

1. anterior/posterior
2. breast self-examination
3. carcinoma *in situ*
4. continuous positive airway pressure
5. dilatation and curettage
6. diethylstilbestrol
7. estrogen replacement therapy
8. fibrocystic breast disease
9. follicle-stimulating hormone
10. gamete-intrafallopian transfer
11. intrauterine device
12. intravenous pyelogram
13. kidneys/ureters/bladder
14. luteinizing hormone
15. pelvic inflammatory disease
16. premenstrual syndrome
17. sexually transmitted disease
18. toxic shock syndrome
19. zygote-intra-fallopian transfer

Self-Assessment Questions

1. a
2. c
3. b
4. a
5. d

Chapter 31　Nursing Care of the Client: Male Reproductive System

Key Terms

1. g
2. d
3. h
4. b
5. j
6. i
7. e
8. a
9. f
10. c

Abbreviation Review

1. American Academy of Pediatrics
2. belladonna and opium
3. benign prostatic hypertrophy
4. breast self-examination
5. diethylstilbestrol
6. dynamic infusion cavernosometry and cavernosography
7. follicle-stimulating hormone
8. luteinizing hormone
9. prostate specific antigen
10. sexually transmitted disease
11. testicular self-examination
12. transurethral ultrasound-guided laser-induced prostatectomy
13. transurethral resection of the prostate
14. urinary tract infection
15. vacuum constriction device

Self-Assessment Questions

1. d
2. b
3. a
4. c
5. d

Chapter 32　Nursing Care of the Client: Sexually Transmitted Diseases

Key Terms

1. e
2. i
3. d
4. f
5. j
6. b
7. g
8. k
9. h
10. a
11. c

Abbreviation Review

1. acquired immunodeficiency syndrome
2. cytomegalovirus
3. enzyme-linked immunosorbent assay
4. hepatitis B virus
5. human immunodeficiency virus
6. human papillomavirus
7. herpes simplex virus
8. pelvic inflammatory disease
9. rapid plasma reagin
10. sexually transmitted disease
11. venereal disease research laboratory

Self-Assessment Questions

1. a
2. a
3. d
4. a
5. c
6. a

Chapter 33　Nursing Care of the Client: Mental Illness

Key Terms

1. m
2. dd
3. mm
4. rr

5. r

6. aa

7. b

8. k

9. v

10. e

11. l

12. gg

13. s

14. f

15. ll

16. ss

17. q

18. cc

19. i

20. bb

21. uu

22. o

23. xx

24. w

25. pp

26. c

27. p

28. ff

29. yy

30. hh

31. x

32. kk

33. g

34. oo

35. bbb

36. qq

37. z

38. j

39. n

40. tt

41. d

42. h

43. ee

44. jj

45. a

46. ii

47. vv

48. u

49. y

50. nn

51. ww

52. zz

53. t

54. aaa

Abbreviation Review

1. attention deficit hyperactivity disorder

2. American Psychiatric Association

3. Adult Protective Services

4. twice a day

5. Child Protective Services

6. *Diagnostic and Statistical Manual of Mental Disorders,* 4th edition

7. electroconvulsive therapy

8. extrapyramidal symptom

9. generalized anxiety disorder

10. intensive care unit

11. monoamine oxidase inhibitor

12. milliequivalents per liter

13. neuroleptic malignant syndrome

14. obsessive compulsive disorder

15. over-the-counter

16. phencyclidine

17. posttraumatic stress disorder

18. selective serotonin reuptake inhibitor

19. tardive dyskinesia

Self-Assessment Questions

1. d

2. a

3. b

4. a

5. d

Chapter 34   Nursing Care of the Client: Substance Abuse

Key Terms

1. d

2. a

3. h

4. j

5. m

6. b

7. n
8. l
9. t
10. i
11. p
12. c
13. o
14. k
15. e
16. g
17. q
18. s
19. r
20. f

Abbreviation Review

1. Alcoholics Anonymous
2. attention deficit hyperactivity disorder
3. alcohol withdrawal syndrome
4. Drug Enforcement Agency
5. diethyltriptamine
6. detoxification
7. dimethyltryptamine
8. dimethyl-4-ethylamphetamine
9. *Diagnostic and Statistical Manual of Mental Disorders,* 4th edition
10. fetal alcohol effects
11. fetal alcohol syndrome
12. lysergic acid diethylamide
13. Mothers Against Drunk Driving
14. monoamine oxidase inhibitor
15. methylenedioxyamphetamine
16. Narcotics Anonymous
17. National Institute on Drug Abuse
18. phencyclidine
19. range of motion
20. Students Against Drunk Driving
21. sudden infant death syndrome

Self-Assessment Questions

1. b
2. c
3. a
4. c
5. a

Chapter 35   Nursing Care of the Older Client

Key Terms

1. c
2. a
3. g
4. j
5. b
6. h
7. f
8. d
9. i
10. e

Abbreviation Review

1. American Association of Retired Persons
2. Alzheimer's disease
3. American Nurses Association
4. Balanced Budget Act
5. benign prostatic hypertrophy
6. congestive heart failure
7. chronic obstructive pulmonary disease
8. estrogen replacement therapy
9. Health Care Financing Agency
10. non-insulin-dependent diabetes mellitus
11. Omnibus Reconciliation Act
12. open reduction/internal fixation
13. prospective payment system
14. prostate specific antigen
15. peripheral vascular disease
16. respiratory tract infection
17. resource utilization group system
18. skilled nursing facility
19. total hip arthoplasty
20. transient ischemic attack
21. urinary tract infection

Self-Assessment Questions

1. b
2. d
3. b
4. c
5. a

Chapter 36 Rehabilitation, Home Health, Long-Term Care, and Hospice

Key Terms

1. c
2. l
3. j
4. b
5. i
6. e
7. k
8. d
9. m
10. a
11. f
12. g
13. n
14. h

Abbreviation Review

1. American Health Care Association
2. Assisted Living Federation of America
3. Commission on Accreditation of Rehabilitation Facilities
4. continuing care retirement community
5. Certification Examination for Practical and Vocational Nurses in Long-Term Care
6. community health accreditation program
7. certified in long-term care
8. extended care facility
9. Health Care Finance Administration
10. health maintenance organization
11. instrumental activities of daily living
12. intermediate care facility
13. interdisciplinary health care team
14. Joint Commission on Accreditation of Healthcare Organizations
15. National Council of State Boards of Nursing
16. Omnibus Budget Reconciliation Act
17. skilled nursing facility

Self-Assessment Questions

1. c
2. a
3. d
4. b
5. c

Chapter 37 Nursing Care of the Client: Responding to Emergencies

Key Terms

1. c
2. a
3. f
4. h
5. b
6. g
7. d
8. i
9. e

Abbreviation Review

1. airway, breathing, circulation
2. cubic centimeter
3. centimeter
4. cardiopulmonary resuscitation
5. emergency department
6. emergency medical services
7. emergency medical technician
8. emergency medical technician—paramedic
9. motor vehicle accident
10. rest, ice, compression, elevation

Self-Assessment Questions

1. a
2. d
3. b
4. d
5. a
6. b